CANADIAN ANGELS OF MERCY: NURSES IN TIMES OF PERIL 1885 - 1918

by
Jasmine Falling Rain Frye
&
J. Wayne Frye

Catalogue Number: 20126196109

ISBN: 978-0-9879728-0-4
Peninsula Publishing
Distributed
by
Fireside Books

Victoria, British Columbia

Table of Contents

Prologue – Page 5
Why Not?
Chapter   1 – Page 8
Healthcare Based on the Profit Motive
Chapter   2 – Page 13
That Little Village Beneath the Snow-Covered
Mesa And Jasmine Frye
Chapter   3 – Page 16
Revered Profession
Chapter   4 - Page 25
Florence Nightingale – Sidney, I Am Sorry
Chapter   5 - Page 71
Georgia Fane Pope: A Women of Deep Compassion
For Those Who Needed It Most
Chapter   6 - Page 79
Mary Meagre Scott: The Florence Nightingale
of Newfoundland
Chapter   7 – Page 87
Ishbel Maria Hamilton-Gordon: In Service to so Many
Who are in Need
Chapter   8 – Page 99
Myra Bennett and the Green House of Mercy
Chapter   9 - Page 102
It Was Our Duty as Canadians
Chapter 10 - Page 136
And the Worst Friend and Enemy is But Death
Chapter 11 - Page 176
They Should be at the Front of the Line
Chapter 12 – Page 187
An Enemy More Deadly Than Any We Saw in the War
Epilogue – Page 193
A More Equalitarian Society
References – Page 197

TO: Dorothy Sullivan, my mother, and, like me, a proud member of the Navajo Nation. *Jasmine Falling Rain Frye*

TO: My sister Dana, who brought great joy to me during a wonderful, but sometimes tumultuous childhood for both of us. *JWF*

ABOUT THE AUTHORS

Wayne Frye is primarily known in Canada as the author of the Aaron Adams mystery novels. However, he has written 12 works of non-fiction, including university textbooks. He has been a university president, university hockey coach, marketing consultant and for over 11 years was director of an intensive academic support program for inner-city children in the Los Angeles area. He moved to Canada in 2003 from the USA and is now a Canadian citizen.

Jasmine Falling Rain Frye is a member of the Navajo Nation. She moved to Canada in 2002, and like her husband, is now a proud Canadian. She studied architecture and interior design at university, and was a housing contractor for many years before deciding to enter the medical field and specialize in Aboriginal care. She and her husband currently reside in Ladysmith (Vancouver Island), British Columbia.

PROLOGUE
WHY NOT?

Ted Kennedy, at his brother Robert's funeral said, "my brother need not be idealized, or enlarged in death beyond what he was in life; to be remembered simply as a good and decent man, who saw wrong and tried to right it, saw suffering and tried to heal it, saw war and tried to stop it."[1]

Those words are particularly apropos to the work of nurses, as they are more than just healers. They are individuals with compassionate natures who work diligently to ameliorate the afflictions, both physical and mental, of those who suffer from disease, war and neglect. In a world that promotes greed as an essential trait to the economic structure of capitalism, compassion is often neglected. Yet, after we are dead, the lavishness of the homes in which we lived, the luxurious cars we drove or the size of our bank accounts will be irrelevant. However, if we have shown compassion toward others, our legacy is forever carved into the psyches of those to whom we gave a helping hand. Hopefully, we will have planted a seed in those we helped that will germinate into compassion they will also show toward others.

For the 99% of us not born into wealth, financial remuneration is a critical component in the consideration of a career path. This does not mean that we are necessarily mercenary human beings. It is simply a necessity in a capitalist system that puts everything from food to communications in the hands of corporations that are always more concerned with the bottom line than compassion. Simple survival in this system necessitates

[1] Ted Kennedy: Eulogy for Robert Kennedy - 1968 - N.Y. Daily News

that we must practice self-perseverance, often at the expense of compassion. However, there are a few professions that offer reasonable financial rewards, but also are the preserve of those who know that compassion is the core of their profession. Nursing is such an endeavour.

There was a time when nursing was considered exclusively a woman's profession, because it was assumed that it was instinctive in a woman's nature to be compassionate and caring. Today, many men are entering the profession, as it is obvious that a compassionate nature is not the exclusive domain of women. However, nursing history is primarily a history of women, simply because of the attractiveness of the profession to that gender at times when it was either considered a career that was unmanly or economically untenable. Obviously, men will be playing more crucial roles in the future of nursing based upon the propensity of them now to consider it as a worthy career.

The nurse has always been a necessity, but until recent times, nurses lacked social status or respect. In primitive times, nurses were slaves, and in more civilized times, considered domestic help. Education was generally lacking, as a nurse was more likely to be considered unskilled worker rather than an educated practitioner with defined medical knowledge.

In the early days of nursing, most skills were not learned in school, but were passed on from one person to another. Nurses were considered menial labourers and expected to obey as any servant would. Denied dignity as a profession, nursing was a magnet for those mired in poverty. Consequently, like today's poor, the nurse was subject to great degradation at the hands of those who felt empowered to use and abuse them. The untrained nurse is as old as the human race, but, fortunately, today's nurses must undergo rigorous education and training before being allowed to practice a profession that puts life and death in their hands every day.

A few nurses and doctors were burned at the stake during the Inquisition, when the church branded some practices heretical. Throughout history, those who promulgated superstition and ignorance, have attempted to stifle medical progress through the imposition of stern admonitions to avoid certain practices that are now considered vital in the administering of competent health care. Human progress is too often slowed by those bound to a past where superstition and dogma tie the hands of those who seek enlightenment. Nurses are a vital element in the battle against human afflictions. To paraphrase Ted Kennedy again: *unlike people who see things as they are and say why, nurses dream things that never were and say why not.*

CHAPTER 1
HEALTHCARE BASED ON THE PROFIT MOTIVE

With the appointment of George Bush as President of the U.S.A. in 2000, seeing no hope for a country that was being turned over to right-wing ideologues and corporations, the authors of this book elected to vote with our feet. In 2002, we were approved for immigration to Canada, and we have never regretted our decision. One of the proudest moments in our lives was when we took the Canadian citizenship oath in 2007.

One of the primary reasons we chose Canada as the place we wanted to immigrate was the simple fact that, unlike the U.S.A., healthcare here is a right, rather than a privilege. Wayne Frye is particularly cognizant of how important it is to guarantee that everyone has access to quality healthcare at no cost. His mother was ill for seven years, and he watched his father's finances being decimated when he had to lay-out 1.2 million dollars for healthcare when his insurance coverage ran out. One time, as his mother was lying on the operating table, his father was forced to count out $80,000 in cash, before the hospital would approve a life-saving operation. This kind of callousness is the reason, that as compassionate human beings, we must fight to make certain that Canadian healthcare is never turned over to the corporations like it has been in the U.S.A.

What does the above have to do with a book about nurses and their contributions to healthcare through the years? Very simply, it is a way of reiterating that as professionals, nurses are a vanguard against privatization that can lead to a corporate executive deciding whether an individual is entitled to certain procedures or not. Nurses must be eternally vigilant as caring professionals to assure that the system of fairness in Canadian healthcare is never abrogated to serve the corporate bottom line. The profit motive has no place in the healthcare equation.

Unfortunately, in the past, nurses have not only had to battle diseases and sicknesses, but struggle valiantly in untenable conditions where health care systems refused care for the less financially fortunate in society by relegating them to substandard facilities. Through war, plagues and other catastrophes, nurses have been selfless adherents for those who suffer. Nurses owe a debt of gratitude to their forbearers who struggled to bring dignity and respect to the profession. We must selflessly continue that struggle to assure that in the future healthcare is considered a human right in every country. All members of society have a special obligation to the poor and vulnerable. The justness of a society is tested by the treatment of the poor, the sick and the disenfranchised. As nurses, we are measured by how the poor, the unprotected, the downtrodden and the stranger receive care. The janitor and the Prime Minister are to be treated no different in our healthcare system. What is good enough for one is good enough for another. The proper administration of quality healthcare can exclude no one. It is within the nurse's purview to speak for the voiceless, to defend the defenceless, to assess life styles, policies, and social institutions in terms of their impact on those for whom we care. This does not mean pitting one group against another, but rather, strengthening the whole community by assisting all with equal compassion and quality of care. The Canadian medical system must never lose sight of these noble goals in assuring healthcare always remains a human right in this country. To this end, one of this book's authors, Wayne Frye, wrote the following article about Canadian healthcare.

It Was a Miracle²
By
J. Wayne Frye

Those of us lucky enough to be Canadians often take our super, world renown health care system for granted. I say that, because I was once a citizen of the United States of America, where healthcare is a privilege, rather than a right.

Mention Tommy Douglas as the man voted the greatest Canadian, and Americans will give you a quizzical look. After all, he was not a Prime Minister, a great general, a hockey player or even much of a politician. Basically, he was just a simple Baptist minister from the prairies of Saskatchewan who one day decided that he could do more for humanity in the halls of the Saskatchewan Legislature than he could in the church pulpit. Today, thanks to his efforts, Canadians enjoy the finest healthcare system in the world and do not have to worry about the costs. His commitment to democratic socialism often led to him being branded a Bolshevik, but he never wavered in his belief that the good of the people should always be the purpose of everything the government does.

A few years after immigrating to Canada, I talked with an old friend from New York City. We had just reconnected after 30 years. When I asked him how his wife was doing, he recounted the story of her battle with cancer and how they had re-mortgaged their house, and he was forced to take a second job and delay retirement to cover the medical expenses not covered by his insurance.

---

² Reprinted with permission from the Canadian Tribune News Syndicate.

I did not have the heart to share with him what I am about to share with you, but I am sharing it with you, so that everyone of my readers can reflect and think about how lucky we are as Canadians to live in a society that is genuinely compassionate and promises that all its citizens will have equal access to the best medical care possible at no cost.

On New Year's Eve, I noticed a mild tingling in my left arm. A week earlier, I had the same feeling when visiting my son in Edmonton, and fortunately, my daughter-in-law, a nurse, insisted that I go to the emergency room immediately. They intonated that I had suffered a mild stroke. In spite of that, as a former American, when the same thing occurred on New Year's Eve, I suppose that old feeling that it would be expensive to go to the emergency room made me insist that I should just wait and go to the doctor's office the next day. Fortunately for me, my wife refused my admonitions to just ignore the pain. She literally pushed me to the car, and we made a quick trip to the local hospital. I must admit that I was scared. We got to the hospital and the parking lot was dark and foreboding. It was midnight. We went through the automatic doors, and the emergency room nurse says, "Oh, it looks like you are in distress, sir. Let me help you."

She put me in a wheelchair, asked about what was wrong and within 30 seconds a doctor had me placed on a gurney. I watched my wife go over to a big oak desk, and I was peering through white curtains, as she asked another person where she made arrangements. I heard the person say, "What do you mean, make arrangements?"

My wife responded, "don't we have to make financial arrangements?"

The nurse smiled and said, "All I need is your Care Card. This is Canada. There are no financial arrangements. Your husband is sick, and he will be taken care of no matter what it costs.

As I laid on the gurney, waiting to be whisked away for tests, I almost cried. I remembered my dad having to put up $80,000 in order for my mother to receive a life-saving operation in the U.S.A., and how he ultimately went through 1.2 million dollars to keep her alive for 7 years. I remembered all the people I knew over the years who had borrowed money or lost homes and businesses to pay for medical care. I thought to myself that Canadians had no idea how lucky they were. To those of us not born into this system, it was a miracle.

Although this book is a compilation of stories about nurses and how they effectuated the development of nursing into one of the most highly respected professions in the world, it is also about how nurses and ordinary citizens, must continue the fight to see that Canadian healthcare never slides into the malaise that is so prevalent in the U.S.A. and the few other countries that cling to an outdated model of healthcare based on the profit motive.

CHAPTER 2
THAT LITTLE VILLAGE BENEATH
THE SNOW-COVERED MESA
AND JASMINE FRYE

Although I am privileged to live in a country where quality healthcare is provided to all citizens at no cost, because of their isolation, many Aboriginal communities are underserved by this system, not because of neglect, but simply because of logistics. For that reason, I elected to devote myself to Aboriginal medical care, particularly for those in isolated places. I wrote the below article when I realized that there was much more that needed to be done to reach out with the hand of compassion to those who live on isolated reserves, rural or remote areas and are underserved by the healthcare system.

THAT LITTLE VILLAGE BENEATH
THE SNOW-COVERED MESA[3]

By
Jasmine Falling Rain Frye

The sky above is obliterated by white, fluffy, mist-filled fog that seems to descend from the heavens and embrace the snow-covered ground upon which I glide effortlessly on my snowmobile. My clinical duties as a First-Nations health professional specializing in aboriginal healthcare take me to isolated areas where there are no roads, but only make-shift trails leading to those few people who still live the way my forefathers did. They are free of the trappings of modern society, some even living without

---

[3] Reprinted with permission from the Canadian Tribune News Syndicate.

electricity or the ever present satellite television dish. My cell-phone only works sporadically, as the signal is often blocked by atmospheric or terrain conditions. Out here in the wilderness, I am at the mercy of the elements and the skill of my snowmobile driver who seems to effortlessly navigate through the majestic snow-laden landscape, as he constantly reminds me to keep a watchful eye on the slid filled with medical supplies we are pulling behind us. This is not a job for the faint-at-heart, but it is a job that I clasp to with great and determined zeal, since it affords me an opportunity to connect with my cultural heritage.

I am one of those aboriginals who was born in the city, but later in life, realized I was a descendant of a noble race of people who had their land stolen and their way of life destroyed by people who considered us savages. To pay homage to my heritage, I have decided to devote the rest of my life in service to Aboriginals who are often shunned by a society that thinks that those who live simply and eschew the ever-prevalent culture of greed are irrelevant in the modern world.

As we drive toward a tall, snow cover mesa, at its base are a row of simple log huts with smoke rising majestically out of ancient stone chimneys. Approaching them, the sounds of our whirring motor bounce off the mesa and reverberate throughout the desolate valley. Within a hundred feet of the huts, we see doors sprang open and people begin to eagerly wave. Our monthly journey to this village offers more than medical assistance. It is a journey of discovery that affords us an opportunity to share in the lives of people who know serenity, peace and tranquility that those of us in so-called civilization can only dream about. These people do not even know it, but they are living in paradise.

The culture of greed that makes us all think that happiness comes with a price tag has no place here. These people welcome us with open arms and gladly share a warm blanket, a cozy seat by the fireplace or a caribou steak. With no need for refrigeration during the winter months, everyone hangs their food in a community storage shed, and gladly shares it with all members of the small village. Hunger or lack of shelter would simply not be tolerated in a society where the pain of one is the pain of all.

After two days of accessing the health of the villagers, as night falls, we mount our snowmobile and head back to what is euphemistically called civilization. The five hour journey will seem tedious as we leave behind a way of life that a few brave souls are fighting desperately to protect from the ever insidious spread of the corporate-based culture that makes slaves of us all. I intend to do all I can as a medical professional to assist in helping these noble people maintain a lifestyle that must be insulated from the cruelties of a society where everything has a price-tag.

Leaving the village far behind, the sound of the roaring engine penetrates the bitterly cold, mist-filled darkness, and I am bewildered as I see the bright lights of the city in the distance. Am I now headed back to civilization, or is the real civilization back in that little village beneath the snow covered mesa?

CHAPTER 3
REVERED PROFESSION

In today's world, nursing is a very popular field of study, and a career as a nurse is becoming more and more demanding. However, it took decades for the profession to actually gain some sort of credit and recognition. It was not until the 19th century that nursing was truly valued, when many remarkable individuals, mostly women, took the stage to find ways to help the wounded and the sick.

Nurses were abused and the job was even used by some authorities as a form of punishment for individuals convicted of crimes during the 17th century. The 20th century saw dramatic changes in nursing as a result of two world wars and the insistence that formalized training be made part of the process. Today, the RN (Registered Nurse) designation means that a nurse has a formal nursing education (usually a Bachelor of Science in Nursing degree – B.Sc.N.) and has passed a rigorous examination before qualifying to practice. Additional designations that require advanced education (Advanced Speciality, M.A. or Ph.D.) include, but are not necessarily limited to the following (Specific Canadian Designations as of 2012 are noted with an *).

*ABORIGINAL CARE:
These nurses' interventions are targeted towards Aboriginal communities and populations. Aboriginal-specific determinants of health, traditional healing, shamanism etc. and Aboriginal values, beliefs and cultures are part of the nursing process.
AMBULATORY CARE:
Ambulatory care nurses care for patients whose stay in the facility will last for less than 24 hours. Ambulatory care

nursing covers a broad range of specialties for the out-patient.

ANESTHESIA:
Nurse Anaesthetists work with surgeons, dentists, podiatrists, anaesthesiologists, and other doctors to provide anaesthesia to patients.

*CARDIOVASCULAR CARE:
The Cardiac Care Nurse works with other members of the medical staff in assessing, intervening, and implementing nursing care for the cardiac patient.

CASE MANAGEMENT:
Case management is a collaborative process of assessment, planning, facilitation and advocacy for options and services to meet an individual's health needs.

*COMMUNITY HEALTH NUSRING:
This nurse conducts a continuing and comprehensive practice that is preventive, curative and rehabilitative. The philosophy of care is based on the belief that care directed to the individual, the family, and the group contributes to the health care of the population as a whole. The community health nurse is not restricted to the care of a particular age or diagnostic group. Participation of all consumers of health care is encouraged in the development of community activities that contribute to the promotion of, education about, and maintenance of good health. These activities require comprehensive health programs that pay special attention to social and ecologic influences and specific populations at risk.

*CRITICAL CARE:
Critical Care nurses provide vital care for patients and families who are experiencing actual or potential life-threatening illnesses. More specific fields that fit into the Critical Care category include Cardiac Care, Intensive Care, and Neurological and Cardiac Surgical Intensive Care.

*CRITICAL CARE PEDIATRIC: Same as above, except applied to the field of pediatrics exclusively.
*EMERGENCY:
Emergency nurses assess patients, provide interventions and evaluate care in a time limited and sometimes hectic environment. These nurses work independently and interdependently with various health professionals in an attempt to support patients and their families as they experience illness, injury or crisis.
*ENTEROSTOMAL THERAPY:
An enterostomal therapy nurse, or ET nurse, has specialized training in treating patients with ostomies (passing stools through an opening cut in the abdomen). An ET nurse may treat patients before, during, and after their ostomy surgery. Some situations that an ET nurse may help with include: Working with patients and surgeons to determine optimal stoma placement, after surgery care, changing the ostomy device and stoma skin care.
FORENSICS:
Forensic nurses provide medical care to victims of crime, collect evidence after crimes occur, and provide medical care to patients within the prison system.
*GASTROENTEROLOGY:
Gastroenterology (GI) nurses provide care to patients with known or suspected gastrointestinal problems who are undergoing diagnostic or therapeutic treatment and/or procedures. GI nurses practice in venues: inpatient and outpatient endoscopy departments, ambulatory endosocopy centres and inpatient hospital units.
*GERONTOLOGICAL:
Gerontological Nursing contributes to and often leads the interdisciplinary and multi-agency care of older people. It may be practiced in a variety of settings although it is most likely to be developed within services or organizations dedicated to the care of older people.

GERIATRICS:
Geriatric nurses care for the elderly in a number of settings which include the patients' homes, nursing homes, and hospitals.

HOLISTIC:
Holistic nurses provide medical care for patients while steadfastly honouring and respecting the individual's subjective opinions about health, health beliefs, cultural heritage and values. Holistic nursing requires nurses to integrate self-care, self-responsibility, spirituality, and reflection.

HIV/AIDS:
HIV/AIDS nurses provide healthcare for patients who are HIV or AIDS positive. These nurses usually have specialized training in HIV/AIDS.

*HOSPICE PALLIATIVE CARE:
Palliative care is the active holistic care of patients with advanced progressive illness. Management of pain and other symptoms and provision of psychological, social and spiritual support is paramount. The goal of palliative care is achievement of the best quality of life for patients and their families

INFORMATICS: Nursing informatics is a broad field which combines nursing knowledge with advanced knowledge of computer modelling.

LEGAL NURSING:
Legal nursing combines the use of the legal system with a thorough knowledge of the nursing field. Legal nurses are usually seasoned veterans of the nursing field who work with attorneys to review medical documents and determine if medical negligence occurred.

*MEDICAL-SURGICAL:
Medical surgical nurses are required to be proficient in all systems of the body: digestive, skeletal, muscular, lymphatic, endocrine, nervous, cardiovascular, reproductive

and urinary. They can work in a hospital, in home care, or in long-term or acute-care facilities. Medical surgical nurses care for and assess patients who recently have had surgery or those who are being treated with pharmaceuticals.

*MIDWIFERY:

Midwives are nurses that are specially trained to deal with childbirth and to providing prenatal and postpartum care. The midwife is qualified to deliver babies by themselves unless there are extenuating circumstances which require the midwife to consult with a physician.

MILITARY:

Military nurses work in a variety of settings, ranging from family practice at a local military base to government settings to providing emergency care for the wounded during war times.

NEONATAL:

Neonatal nurses provide care for newborns by assessing the patient to ensure good health, providing preventative care to prevent illness, and caring for the babies which are sick. The neonatal nurse is responsible for anticipating, preventing, diagnosing and minimizing illnesses of newborns.

*NEPHROLOGY:

Nephrology nurses deal with chronic kidney disease that damages the kidneys, allowing wastes to build in the blood and failing to maintain proper blood pressure.

*NURSE PRACTITIONER:

Nurse practitioners are advanced practice nurses who have obtained their masters degree and are qualified to prescribe medication, and interpret diagnostic and laboratory tests in a variety of settings.

*NEUROSCIENCE:

These nurses care for patients using new therapies and innovative technologies to treat diseases of the nervous

system.
*OCCUPATIONAL HEALTH:
Occupational Health Nursing is responsible for improving, protecting, maintaining and restoring the health of employees. By providing this care for employees, the occupational health nurse influences the health of the organization.
*ONCOLOGY:
Oncology nurses provide health care for cancer patients at all stages of treatment and remission.
*ORTHOPAEDIC:
A nurse whose primary area competence and professional practice is the branch of nursing concerned with the prevention and correction of disorders of the locomotor system, including the skeleton, muscles, joints, and related tissues.
PEDIATRIC:
Pediatric nurses care for children in all aspects of health care. Pediatric nurses practice in a variety of settings which include hospitals, clinics, schools, and in the home.
*PERINATAL:
(Also See Neonatal) The perinatal period is the period "around birth," meaning the time of pregnancy, birth, and the first few days or weeks of life as a new or growing family. This is a vulnerable and powerful time for the mother, the fetus, and the family. Perinatal clinical nurse specialists help meet the essential maternal and fetal health needs during this crucial time for the family's long-term health and well being.
*PERIOPERATIVE (OR):
Perioperative nurses work in operating rooms in tertiary care hospitals, community and rural hospitals, day care surgery units and highly specialized clinics in a variety of locations and venues. They provide post-anesthetic patient care in rural hospitals or specialized patient units.

*PSYCHIATRIC/MENTAL HEALTH:
Psychiatric nurses provide specified care for patients and families with defined psychiatric or mental illnesses.
*REHABILITATION:
Rehabilitation nurses help individuals affected by chronic illness or physical disability to adapt to their disabilities, achieve their greatest potential and work toward productive, independent lives.
RESEARCH:
Research nurses perform clinical and basic research to establish a scientific basis for the care of individuals across the life span from management of patients during illness and recovery to the reduction of risks for disease and disability, the promotion of healthy lifestyles, promoting quality of life in those with chronic illness, and care for those individuals at the end of life.
SCHOOL NURSING:
School nurses work with students and faculty of schools providing medical care and other support in an in-school environment.
TRANSPLANT:
Transplant nurses work in a variety of settings and function in various aspects of transplant procedures. They assist in the transplantation of various body parts which include, but are not limited to the liver, kidney, pancreas, small bowel, heart and lungs.
TRAUMA:
Trauma nurses care for patients in an emergency or critical care setting. These nurses generally care for patients who have suffered severe trauma such as a car accident, gun shot wound, stabbing, assault, or other traumatic injury.
TRAVEL NURSING:
hospitals and other health care facilities across the country. Travel nurses usually get to choose which locations they

are willing to travel to and are typically given assignments which last for 13 weeks or more. Travel nurses usually, in addition to a good salary, receive paid housing accommodations, sign-on bonuses, and other ancillary benefits.

UROLOGY:

Urology nurses care for patients in such specialties as oncology, male infertility, male sexual dysfunction, kidney stones, incontinence, and pediatrics. Urology nurses may also participate in urological surgeries for cancer, general urology, infertility, brachytherapy, lithotripsy, and pediatric surgery.

WOMEN'S HEALTH:

Women's health nurses participate in fields such as OB/GYN, mammography, reproductive health, and general women's health. These nurses practice in a variety of settings.[4]

There are nursing shortages all over the world, and they are predicted to become more pronounced in the future. As the world continues to recognize the immense value of this profession, it is incumbent upon those who are either in the field, or are planning on entering it, to make sure that they realize the dept of gratitude owed to the many nurses who have worked hard to make it an honourable and respected profession. The purpose of this book is to pay homage to a few brave, pioneering nurses who worked diligently to make this an honoured, respected and revered profession.

---

[4] Retrieved from http://www.allnurses.com and http://www.cna-nurses/specialities.aspx

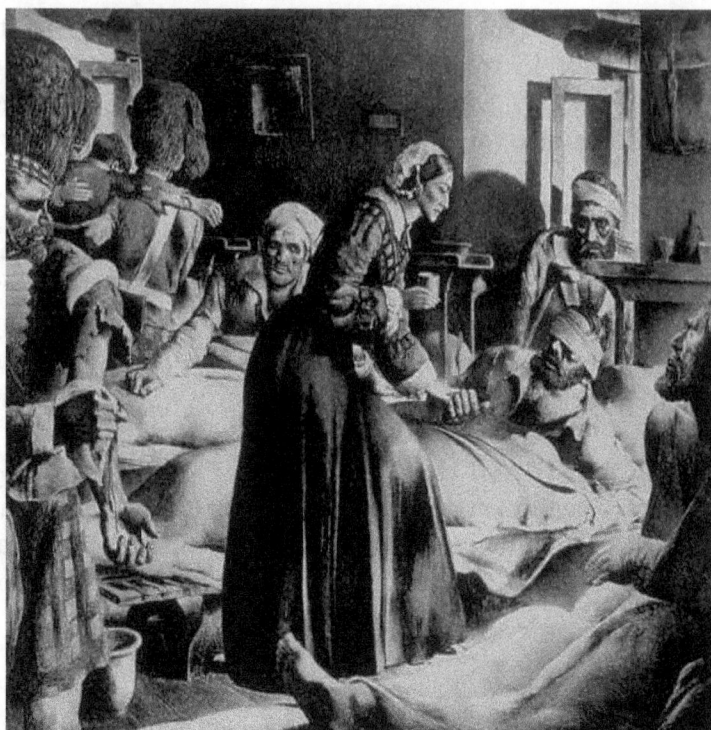

FLORENCE NIGHTINGALE TENDING TO SOLDIERS
DURING THE CRIMEAN WAR[5]

Florence Nightingale laid the foundation of professional nursing with the establishment, in 1860, of her nursing school at St Thomas' Hospital in London, the first secular nursing school in the world, now part of King's College London. The Nightingale Pledge taken by new nurses was named in her honour, and the annual International Nurses Day is celebrated around the world on her birthday.[6]

---

[5] Retrieved from http:/www.gardenofpraise.com/ibdnight.htm
[6] Retrieved from http//www.wikipedia.org/wiki/Florence_Nightingale

CHAPTER 4
FLORENCE NIGHTINGALE – "SIDNEY, I AM SORRY"

Although not Canadian, no book on nurses can exclude Florence Nightingale. Nursing was traditionally a career for young women, in a time when most other careers were not an option. Many famous nurses in history were young women who wanted to be more than wives and mothers. One of the most unlikely women to be a nurse was Florence Nightingale. Yet, today, she is the standard by which all nurses are judged.

Florence Nightingale was born in 1820 into a rich British family. Her determination to become a nurse seemed foolish and crazy, because at this time, nursing was very much seen as a lower-class pursuit. Nurses were given very little training, and hospitals were viewed with fear as the place people went to die. Florence would not be deterred, however, and trained at the Institute of Protestant Deaconesses at Kaiserswerth, in Germany, becoming a nurse in 1851.[7]

Let us now take a look at an extraordinary woman whose name has become synonymous with nursing.

Eminent Victorians – Florence Nightingale in the Age of Reason [8]

Everyone knows the popular conception of Florence Nightingale. The saintly, self-sacrificing woman, the

---

[7] Retrieved from http://www.licensedpracticalnurse.org/famous-nurses
[8] Frye, J. & Lytton, S.. (2011) Eminent Victorians with Correctional Accuracy from 1918.

delicate maiden of high degree who threw aside the pleasures of a life of ease to succour the afflicted, the lady with the lamp, gliding through the horrors of the hospital at Scutari, and consecrating with the radiance of her goodness the dying soldier's couch, the vision is familiar to all who study history., but the truth was different. The Miss Nightingale of fact was not as facile fancy painted her. She worked in another fashion, and towards another end, she moved under the stress of an impetus which finds no place in the popular imagination as a demon possessed her. Now demons, whatever else they may be, are full of interest. And so it happens that in the real Miss Nightingale there was more that was interesting than in the legendary one, and there was also less that was agreeable.

Her family was extremely well-to-do, and connected by marriage with a spreading circle of other well-to-do families. There was a large country house in Derbyshire; there was another in the New Forest; there were Mayfair Hotel rooms for the London season and all its finest parties; there were tours on the continent with even more than the usual number of Italian operas and of glimpses at the celebrities of Paris. Brought up among such advantages, it was only natural to suppose that Florence would show a proper appreciation of them by doing her duty in that state of by marrying, after a fitting number of dances and dinner-parties, an eligible gentleman, and living happily ever afterwards. Her sister, her cousins, all the young ladies of her acquaintance, were either getting ready to do this or had already done it. It was inconceivable that Florence should dream of anything else; yet dream she did. What was that secret voice in her ear, if it was not a call? Why had she felt, from her earliest years, those mysterious promptings towards non-conventionality. Why, as a child in the nursery, when her sister had shown a healthy pleasure in tearing her dolls to pieces, had she shown an almost morbid one in sewing them up again? Why was she driven now to minister to the poor in their cottages, to watch by sick-beds, to put her dog's wounded paw into elaborate splints as if it was a human being? Why was her head filled with queer imaginations of the family's country house at Embley turned, by some enchantment, into a hospital, with herself as matron moving about among the beds? Why was even her vision of heaven itself filled with suffering patients to whom she was being useful? So she dreamed and wondered, and, taking out her diary, she poured into it the agitations of her soul.

As the years passed, a restlessness began to grow upon her. She was unhappy, and at last she knew it. Mrs. Nightingale, too, began to notice that there was something wrong. Her father suggested that a husband might be advisable; but the curious thing was that she seemed to take no interest in husbands. And with her attractions, and her accomplishments, too. There was nothing in the world to prevent her making a really brilliant match. But no, she would think of nothing but how to satisfy that singular craving of hers to be doing something she considered valuable to humanity.

Florence's mother could not understand her daughter's penchant for doing the unconventional, and then one day her perplexity was changed to consternation and alarm. Florence announced an extreme desire to go to Salisbury Hospital for several months as a nurse; and she confessed to some visionary plan of eventually setting up in a house of her own in a neighbouring village, and there founding "something like a Protestant Sisterhood, without vows, for women of educated feelings." The whole scheme was summarily brushed aside as preposterous; and Mrs.

Nightingale, after the first shock of terror, was able to settle down again more or less comfortably to her embroidery. But Florence, who was now twenty-five and felt that the dream of her life had been shattered, came near to desperation.

And, indeed, the difficulties in her path were great. For not only was it an almost unimaginable thing in those days for a woman of means to make her own way in the world and to live in independence, but the particular profession for which Florence was clearly marked out both by her instincts and her capacities was at that time a peculiarly disreputable one. A "nurse" meant then a coarse old woman, always ignorant, usually dirty, often brutal, in bunched-up sordid garments, tippling at the brandy-bottle or indulging in worse irregularities. The nurses in the hospitals were especially notorious for immoral conduct; sobriety almost unknown among them; and they could hardly be trusted to carry out the simplest medical duties. Certainly, things have changed since those days; and that they have changed is due, far more than to any other human being, to Miss Nightingale herself. It is not to be wondered at that her parents should have shuddered at the notion of their daughter devoting her life to such an occupation. "It was as if," she herself said afterwards, "I had wanted to be a kitchen-maid." Yet, the want, absurd, impracticable as it was, not only remained fixed immovably in her heart, but grew in intensity day by day. Her wretchedness deepened into a morbid melancholy.

A weaker spirit would have been overwhelmed by the load of such distresses, would have yielded or snapped. But this extraordinary young woman held firm, and fought her way to victory. With an amazing persistency, during the eight years that followed her rebuff over Salisbury

Hospital, she struggled and worked and planned. While superficially she was carrying on the life of a brilliant girl in high society, while internally she was a prey to the tortures of regret and of remorse, she yet possessed the energy to collect the knowledge and to undergo the experience which alone could enable her to do what she had determined she would do in the end. In secret she devoured the reports of medical commissions, the pamphlets of sanitary authorities, the histories of hospitals and homes. She spent the intervals of the London season in ragged schools and workhouses. When she went abroad with her family, she used her spare time so well that there was hardly a great hospital in Europe with which she was not acquainted, hardly a great city whose slums she had not passed through. She managed to spend some days in a convent school in Rome, and some weeks as a "Sœur de Charité" in Paris. Then, while her mother and sister were enjoying the restorative waters at Carlsbad, she succeeded in slipping off to a nursing institution at Kaiserswerth, where she remained for more than three months. This was the critical event of her life. The experience she gained as a nurse at Kaiserswerth formed the foundation of all her future action and finally fixed her in her career.

Yet, one other trial awaited her. The allurements of the world she had brushed aside with disdain and loathing; she had resisted the subtler temptation which, in her weariness, had sometimes come upon her, of devoting her baffled energies to art or literature; the last ordeal appeared in the shape of a desirable young man. Up to this point, her many lovers had been nothing to her but an added burden and a mockery. For a moment, she wavered. A new feeling swept over her, a feeling which she had never known before, which she was never to know again. The most powerful and the profoundest of all the instincts of humanity laid claim upon her. It rose before her that instinct for the inevitable habiliments of a Victorian marriage; and she had the strength to stamp it underfoot. She looked at her beloved and said, "I have an intellectual nature which requires satisfaction and that I would find in you. I have a passionate nature which requires satisfaction, and that would I find in you. I have a moral, an active nature which requires satisfaction, and that I would not find in you. Sometimes I think that I will satisfy my passionate nature at all events, but then I think about my moral responsibilities to those who suffer and relent." Thus ended her last flirtation with marriage.

Three years passed, and then at last her family seemed to realize that she was old enough and strong enough to have her way, and she became the superintendent of a charitable nursing home on Harley Street in London. She had gained her independence, though it was in a meagre sphere, and her mother was still not quite resigned and would share with her intimates the oft repeated, "we are ducks who have hatched a wild swan." Florence's mother was wrong. It was not a swan they had hatched. It was an eagle who would soar to great heights.

Nightingale had been a year in her nursing-home in Harley Street, when fate knocked at the door. The Crimean War broke out; the battle of the Alma was fought; and the terrible condition of the military hospitals at Scutari, Turkey began to be known in England. It sometimes happens that all the stars line-up in a favourable array and this was one of those times where there was a perfect configuration of events. For years Miss Nightingale had been getting ready for something momentous, though she did not know what. She was thirty-four, desirous to serve, and the Crimean War afforded her that opportunity. If the war had fallen a few years earlier, she would have lacked the knowledge, perhaps even the power, for such work; a few years later and she would, no doubt, have been fixed in the routine of some absorbing task, and moreover, she would have been growing old. Nor was it only the coincidence of time that was remarkable. It so fell out that Sidney Herbert was at the War Office and in the Cabinet; and Sidney Herbert was an intimate friend of Miss Nightingale's, convinced, from personal experience in charitable work, of her supreme capacity. After such premises, it seems hardly more than a matter of course that her letter, in which she offered her services for the East, and Sidney Herbert's letter, in which he asked for them, should actually have crossed in the post. Thus it all happened, without a hitch. The appointment was made, and even Florence's mother, overawed by the magnitude of the venture, could only approve. A pair of faithful friends offered themselves as personal attendants; thirty-eight nurses were collected; and within a week of the crossing of the letters Miss Nightingale, amid a great burst of popular enthusiasm, left for Constantinople (now Istanbul, Turkey).[9]

As dark had been the picture of the state of affairs at Scutari, revealed to the English public in the despatches of the *London Times* correspondent and in a multitude of private letters, the reality turned out to be darker still. What had occurred was, in brief, the complete break-down of the medical arrangements at the seat of war. The origins of this awful failure were complex and manifold; they stretched back through long years of peace and carelessness in England; they could be traced through endless ramifications of administrative incapacity, from the

---

[9] Retrieved from http:www.en.wikipedia.org/wiki/Florence_ Nightingale

inherent faults of confused systems to the petty bungling of minor officials, from the inevitable ignorance of Cabinet Ministers to the fatal exactitudes of narrow routine. In the inquiries which followed it was clearly shown that the evil was in reality that worst of all evils, one which has been caused by nothing in particular and for which no one in particular was to blame. The whole organization of the war machine was incompetent and out of date. Thus the most obvious precautions were neglected, the most necessary preparations put off from day to day. The principal medical officer of the army, Dr. Hall, was summoned from India at a moment's notice, and was unable to visit England before taking up his duties at the front. The war had raged for many months, before a hospital accommodation at Scutari was acquired for more than a thousand men. Errors, follies, and vices on the part of individuals there and the enormous calamity of administrative collapse was evident everywhere. Into this monstrous, calamitous situation came Florence Nightingale.

Miss Nightingale arrived at Scutari, a suburb of Constantinople (now Istanbul, Turkey), on the Asiatic side of the Bosporus Straits—on November 4th, 1854. It was ten days after the battle of Balaclava, and the day before the battle of Inkerman. The organization of the hospitals, which had already given way under the stress of the battle of the Alma, was now to be subjected to the further pressure which these two desperate and bloody engagements implied. Great detachments of wounded were already beginning to pour in. The men, after receiving such summary treatment as could be given them at the smaller hospitals in the Crimea itself, were forthwith shipped in batches of two hundred across the Black Sea to Scutari. This voyage was in normal times one of four days and a half, but the times were no longer normal, and now the transit often lasted for a fortnight or three weeks. Men who had just undergone the amputation of limbs, men in the clutches of fever or of frostbite, men in the last stages of dysentery and cholera were without beds, sometimes without blankets, often hardly clothed. The one or two surgeons on board did what they could, but medical stores were lacking, and the only form of nursing available was that provided by a handful of invalid soldiers, who were usually themselves prostrate by the end of the voyage. There was no other food beside the ordinary salt rations of ship diet; and even the water was sometimes in short supply. For many months, the average of deaths during these voyages was seventy-four in a thousand. The corpses were unceremoniously hurled overboard.

At Scutari, the landing dock could only be approached with great difficulty, and, in rough weather, not at all. When it was reached, what remained of the men in the ships had first to be disembarked, and then conveyed up a steep slope to the nearest of the hospitals. The most serious cases might be put upon stretcher, as there were far too few for all. The rest were carried or dragged up the hill by ambulatory soldiers who were not too obviously infirm for work. One by one, living or dying, the wounded were carried up into the hospital. And in the hospital what did they find there?   The delusive doors bore no inscription, but it could have simply said "welcome to hell."

Want, neglect, confusion, misery, in every shape and in every degree of intensity, filled the endless corridors and the vast apartments of the gigantic barrack-house, which, without forethought or preparation, had been hurriedly set aside as the chief shelter for the victims of the war. The very building itself was radically defective. Huge sewers underlay it, and cess-pools loaded with filth wafted their poison into the upper rooms. The floors were in so rotten a condition that many of them could not be scrubbed, the walls were thick with dirt; incredible multitudes of vermin swarmed everywhere. Enormous as the building was, it was yet too small. It contained seven kilometres of beds, crushed together so close that there was but just room to pass between them. Under such conditions, the most elaborate system of ventilation might well have been at fault; but here there was no ventilation. The stench was indescribable. "I have been well acquainted," said Miss Nightingale, "with the dwellings of the worst parts of most of the great cities in Europe, but have never been in any atmosphere which I could compare with that of the Barrack Hospital at night." The structural defects were equalled by the deficiencies in the commonest objects of hospital use. There were not enough bedsteads, and the sheets were of canvas, and so coarse that the wounded men recoiled from them, begging to be left in their blankets. There was no bedroom furniture of any kind, and empty beer-bottles were used for candlesticks. There were no basins, no towels, no soap, no brooms, no mops, no trays, no plates. There were neither slippers nor scissors and no knives, forks or spoons. The supply of fuel was constantly deficient. The cooking arrangements were preposterously inadequate, and the laundry was a farce. As for purely medical materials, the tale was no better. Stretchers, splints, bandages were all were lacking; and so were the most ordinary drugs.

To replace such wants, to struggle against such difficulties, there was a handful of men overburdened by the strain of ceaseless work, bound down by the traditions of official routine, and enfeebled either by old age or inexperience or sheer incompetence. They had proved utterly unequal to their task. The principal doctor was lost in the imbecilities of a senile optimism. The wretched official whose business it was to provide for the wants of the hospital was tied fast hand and foot by red tape. A few of the younger doctors struggled valiantly, but what could they do? Unprepared, disorganised, with such help only as they could find among the miserable band of convalescent soldiers drafted off to tend their sick comrades, they were faced with disease, mutilation, and death in all its most appalling forms, crowded multitudinously about them in an ever increasing mass. They were like men in a shipwreck, fighting, not for safety, but for the next moment's bare existence to gain, by yet another frenzied effort, some brief respite from the waters of destruction.

In these surroundings, those who had been long inured to scenes of human suffering found a depth of horror which they had never known before. There were moments, there were places, in the Barrack Hospital at Scutari, where the strongest hand was struck with trembling, and the boldest eye would turn away its gaze.

Miss Nightingale came, and she, at any rate, in that hell, did not abandon hope. Before she left London she had consulted Dr. Andrew Smith, the head of the Army Medical Board, as to whether it would be useful to take out stores of any kind to Scutari; and Dr. Andrew Smith had told her that "nothing was needed." Others had given her similar assurances. Yet, she preferred to trust her own instincts, and at Marseilles, France purchased a large quantity of miscellaneous provisions, which were of the utmost use at Scutari. She came, too, amply provided with money, as she had procured huge donations from private sources, and in addition, she was able to avail herself of another valuable means of help. At the same time as herself, Mr. Macdonald, of the *London Times,* had arrived at Scutari, charged with the duty of administering the large sums of money collected through the agency of that newspaper in aid of the sick and wounded. Mr. Macdonald had the sense to see that the best use he could make of the *Times* Fund was to put it at the disposal of Miss Nightingale. After three weeks watching Florence's work, MacDonald cabled back to London the following:

"I cannot conceive as I now calmly look back on the first three weeks after the arrival of the wounded from Inkerman, how it could have been possible to have avoided a state of things too disastrous to contemplate had not Miss Nightingale been here."

This dispatch was appalling to those who were responsible for the deplorable conditions, and they did not look kindly on this society woman who had decided to become a nurse. Anyway, nurses were no better than scrub women to the men who ran the British Army. With such a frame of mind in the highest quarters, it is easy to imagine the kind of disgust and alarm with which the sudden intrusion of a band of amateurs and females must have filled the minds of the ordinary officer and the ordinary military surgeon. They could not understand it; what had women to do with war? One surgeon, Dr. Hall, an exceedingly arrogant man, who had curried favour to worm his way to the top of his profession, was struck speechless with astonishment at Florence's lack of probity, and at last said, "Miss Nightingale's appointment was extremely droll and unneeded."

Her position was, indeed, an official one, but it was hardly the easier for that. In the hospitals it was her duty to provide the services of herself and her nurses when they were asked for by the doctors, and not until then. At first, some of the surgeons would have nothing to say to her, and, though she was welcomed by others, the majority were hostile and suspicious. However, gradually she gained ground. Her good will could not be denied, and her capacity could not be disregarded. With consummate tact, with all the gentleness of supreme strength, she managed at last to impose her personality upon the susceptible, overwrought, discouraged, and helpless group of men in authority who surrounded her. She stood firm as a rock in a sea of despair, offering those who suffered safety, comfort and life.

So it was that hope dawned at Scutari. The reign of chaos and old way of doing things began to dwindle; order came upon the scene, and common sense, and forethought, and decision, radiating out from the little room off the great gallery in the Barrack Hospital where day and night, the Lady Superintendent was at her task. Progress might be slow, but it was sure. The first sign of a great change came with the appearance of some of those necessary objects the hospitals had been denied for months. The sick men began to enjoy the use of towels and soap, knives and forks, combs and tooth-brushes. Dr. Hall might snort when he heard of it, asking, with a growl, what a soldier wanted with a tooth-brush; but the good work went on. Eventually the whole business of purveying to the hospitals was, in effect, carried out by Miss Nightingale. She alone, it seemed, whatever the contingency, knew where to lay her hands on what was wanted. She alone could dispense her stores with readiness, as above all she alone possessed the art of circumventing the pernicious influences of official etiquette. This was her greatest enemy, and sometimes even she was baffled by it. On one occasion, 27,000 shirts sent out at her instance by the Home Government arrived, were landed, and were only waiting to be unpacked. But the official quartermaster in charge of supplies intervened; "he could not unpack them," he said, "without Board approval."

Florence pleaded hopelessly while the ailing and wounded soldiers lay half-naked shivering for want of clothing. Three weeks of bureaucratic delays elapsed before the shirts were released. A little later, however, on a similar occasion, Miss Nightingale felt that she could assert her own authority. She ordered a government consignment to be forcibly opened, while the miserable quartermaster stood by, wringing his hands in disgust that a woman would usurp his authority.

Vast quantities of valuable stores sent from England lay, she found, engulfed in the bottomless abyss of the Turkish Customs House. Other ship-loads, buried beneath munitions of war destined for Balaclava, passed Scutari without a sign, and thus hospital materials were sometimes carried to and fro three times over the Black Sea before they reached their destination. The whole system was clearly at fault, and Miss Nightingale suggested to the home authorities that a Government Store House should be instituted at Scutari for the reception and distribution of the consignments. Six months after her arrival, this was done by reluctant authorities who still felt that women should have no authority in any British institution.

In the meantime Florence had reorganized the kitchens and the laundries in the hospitals. The ill-cooked hunks of meat, vilely served at irregular intervals, which had hitherto been the only diet for the sick men were replaced by punctual meals, well-prepared and appetizing, while strengthening extra foods like soups, wines, and jellies ("preposterous luxuries," snarled Dr. Hall) were distributed to those who needed them. One thing, however, she could not effect. The separation of the bones from the meat was no part of official cookery, as the rule was that the food must be divided into equal portions, and if some of the portions were all bone - well, every man must take his chance. The rule, perhaps, was not a very good one; but there it was. "It would require a new regulation of the service," she was told, "to bone the meat." As for the washing arrangements, they were revolutionized. Up to the time of Miss Nightingale's arrival the number of shirts which the authorities had succeeded in washing was seven. The hospital bedding, she found, was "washed" in cold water. She took a Turkish house, had boilers installed, and employed soldiers' wives to do the laundry work. The expenses were defrayed from her own funds and that of the *London Times,* and henceforward the sick and wounded had the comfort of clean linen.

Then she turned her attention to the soldiers' clothing. Owing to military exigencies, most men had abandoned their issued clothing. Their knapsacks were lost in battle and they possessed nothing but the clothing they had on when brought to the hospital. The quartermaster, of course, pointed out that, according to the regulations, all soldiers should bring with them into hospital an adequate supply of clothing, and he declared that it was no business of his to make good their deficiencies. Apparently, it was the business of Miss Nightingale. She procured socks, boots, and shirts in enormous quantities. She had trousers made. She rigged up dressing-gowns. "The fact is," she told one of her nurses, "I am now clothing the British Army."

All at once, word came from the Crimea that a great new contingent of sick and wounded might shortly be expected. Where were they to go? Every available corner of the wards was occupied. There were some dilapidated rooms in the Barrack Hospital, unfit for human habitation, but Miss Nightingale believed that if measures were promptly taken they might be made capable of accommodating several hundred beds. One of the doctors agreed with her; the rest of the officials were irresolute, as it would be a very expensive job that would involve building, and who could take the responsibility? The proper course was that a representation should be made to the Director-General of the Army Medical Department in London, then the Director-General would apply to the Finance Office. The Finance Office would apply to the Ordnance Department and the Ordnance Department would lay the matter before the Treasury, and, if the Treasury gave its consent, the work might be correctly carried through, several months after the necessity for it had disappeared.

Watching all the suffering around here, Miss Nightingale, however, had made up her mind that time was of the essence, and she persuaded a British Admiralty Lord, or thought she had persuaded him, to give his sanction to the required expenditure. A hundred and twenty-five workmen were immediately engaged, and the work was begun. The workmen struck over working for a woman, whereupon the Lord washed his hands of the whole business. Miss Nightingale engaged two hundred other workmen on her own authority, and paid the bill out of her own resources. The wards were ready by the required date. Five hundred sick men were received in them, and all the utensils, including knives, forks, spoons, cans and towels, were supplied by Miss Nightingale.

This remarkable woman was in truth performing the function of an administrative chief. How had this come about? Was she not in reality merely a nurse? Was it not her duty simply to tend to the sick? And indeed, was it not as a ministering angel, a gentle "lady with a lamp" that she actually impressed the minds of her contemporaries? No doubt that was so; and yet it is no less certain that, as she herself said, the specific business of nursing was "the least important of the functions into which she had been forced." It was clear that in the state of disorganization into which the hospitals at Scutari had fallen the most pressing, the really vital, need was for something more than nursing; it was for the necessary elements of civilized life - the commonest material objects, the most ordinary cleanliness, the rudimentary habits of order and authority.

For to those who watched her at work among the sick, moving day and night from bed to bed, with that unflinching courage, with that indefatigable vigilance, it seemed as if the concentrated force of an undivided and unparalleled devotion could hardly suffice for that portion of her task alone. Wherever, in those vast wards, suffering was at its worst and the need for help was greatest, there, as if by magic, was Miss Nightingale. Her superhuman equanimity would, at the moment of some ghastly operation, give the victim to courage to endure and hope. Her sympathy would assuage the pangs of dying and bring back to those still living something of the forgotten charm of life. Over and over again her untiring efforts rescued those whom the surgeons had abandoned as beyond the possibility of cure. Her mere presence brought with it a strange influence. A passionate idolatry spread among the men. They kissed her shadow as it passed. They did more. "Before she came," said a soldier, "there was cussing and swearing, but after that it was as 'holy as a church.'"

To the wounded soldiers on their beds of agony she might well appear in the guise of a gracious angel of mercy, but the military surgeons, and the orderlies, and her own nurses could tell a different story. It was not by gentle sweetness and angelic countenance that she had brought order out of chaos, but rather, it was by strict method, stern discipline, rigid attention to detail, ceaseless labour and the fixed determination of an indomitable will. Beneath her cool and calm demeanour lurked fierce and passionate fires. As she passed through the wards in her plain dress, so quiet, so unassuming, she struck the casual observer simply as the pattern of a perfect lady; but the keener eye perceived something more than that. It was the serenity of high deliberation in the scope of the capacious brow, the sign of power in the dominating curve of the thin nose, and the traces of a harsh and dangerous temper, sometimes peevish, sometimes mocking, and yet something precise. There was a smile on her face of the most pleasant kind, but beneath that calm demeanour was a furious advocate for those who suffered.

As for her voice, it was soft and melodic, never raised in anger, but determined in nature. When she had spoken, it seemed as if nothing could follow but obedience. Once, when she had given some direction, a doctor ventured to remark that the thing could not be done. "But it must be done," said Miss Nightingale. A chance bystander, who heard the words, never forgot through all his life the irresistible authority of her quietly, softly spoken words.

Late at night, when the vast number of beds lay wrapped in darkness, Miss Nightingale would sit at work in her little room, over her correspondence. It was one of the most formidable of all her duties. There were hundreds of letters to be written to the friends and relations of soldiers, there was the enormous mass of official documents to be dealt with, there were her own private letters to be answered, and most important of all, there was the composition of her long and confidential reports to Sidney Herbert. These were by no means official communications. Her soul, pent up all day in the restraint and reserve of a vast responsibility, now at last poured itself out in these letters with all its natural vehemence, like a swollen torrent of water sweeping over rapids. Here, at least, she did not mince matters. Here she painted in her darkest colours the hideous scenes which surrounded her. She tore away remorselessly the last veils still shrouding the abominable truth. Then she would fill pages with recommendations and suggestions, with criticisms of the inflexibility of those in charge, with elaborate calculations of contingencies, with exhaustive analyses and statistical statements piled up in breathless eagerness one on the top of the other. And then her pen, in the virulence of its volubility, would rush on to the discussion of individuals, to the denunciation of an incompetent surgeon or the ridicule of an in-sufficient nurse. Her sarcasm searched the ranks of the officials with the deadly and unsparing precision of a machine-gun. Her nicknames were terrible. She respected no one, as she railed against them all. The intolerable futility of mankind obsessed her like a nightmare, and she cried out in anger against the well-being of those she served.

Public opinion in England early recognized the high importance of her mission, and its enthusiastic appreciation of her work soon reached an extraordinary height. The Queen herself was deeply moved. She made repeated inquiries as to the welfare of Miss Nightingale and she asked to see her accounts of the wounded, and made her the intermediary between the throne and the troops.

In May, 1855, after six months of labour, Miss Nightingale could look with something like satisfaction at the condition of the Scutari hospitals. Had the soldiers done nothing more than survive the terrible strain which had been put upon them, it would have been amazing, but they had done much more than that as the loving care they received from Florence and her nurses lifted their spirits and gave them the courage to struggle against formidable odds. The confusion and the pressure in the wards had come to an end. Order reigned in them, cleanliness prevailed and the supplies were bountiful and prompt.

One simple comparison of figures revealed the extraordinary change. The rate of mortality among the cases treated fell from 42% to 2.2%.[10] Still, the indefatigable lady was not satisfied. The main problem had been solved as the physical needs of the men had been provided for, but she was also concerned with their mental and spiritual needs. She set up and furnished reading-rooms and recreation-rooms. She started classes and lectures. Officers were amazed to see her treating their men as if they were human beings, and assured her that she would only end by "spoiling the brutes." But that was not Miss Nightingale's opinion as she became a banker for the soldiers, receiving and sending home large sums of money every month. At last, reluctantly, the Government followed suit, and established machinery of its own for the remission of money. Although to this day, the officer class continues to receive preferential treatment in most armies all over the world, thanks to the efforts of people like Florence Nightingale, they are no longer treated with complete disrespect and little regard for their welfare. She saw that those who did most of the fighting and dying were from the lower socio-economic classes, but she felt that they deserved equal treatment when wounded to that received by

---

[10] Retrieved from http://www.agnescott.edu/lriddle/women/miegale. htm

their superiors. Although this was never completely realized at the time, she fought valiantly for the rights of all to receive equal medical treatment. This battle continues today in a world where social class far too often plays a role in the medical care an individual receives. Even in the equality-based Canadian medical system, those with wealth and power often refuse to wait for services like everyone else must, so they take flight to the U.S.A. to receive treatment in a system where the profit motive allows catering to those with money and power at the expense of the less fortunate. In a very real sense, Florence Nightingale was a soul-mate to the beloved father of Canadian Medicare, Tommy Douglas, because she fervently believed that everyone, regardless of station in life, deserved competent, compassion medical care free of charge.

Amid all these activities, Miss Nightingale took up the further task of inspecting the hospitals in the Crimea itself. The labour was extreme, and the conditions of life were almost intolerable. She spent whole days on horseback or was driven over bleak and rocky heights in a baggage cart. Sometimes she stood for hours in the heavily falling snow, and would only reach her hut at dead of night after walking many kilometres through perilous ravines. Her powers of resistance seemed incredible, but at last they were exhausted. She was attacked by fever, and for a moment came very near death. Yet, she worked on. When she was strong enough to travel, she was ordered back to England, but she steadfastly refused. She would not go back, she said, before the last of the soldiers had left Scutari.

Dr. Hall's labours had been rewarded by a Knighthood; and henceforth, he was to be Sir John. Miss Nightingale told Sidney Herbert, she could only suppose Sir John to be the "Knight of the Crimean Burial-grounds," due to his incompetence. However, he was now Sir John, and he would be thwarted no longer. His determination to rid himself of Florence was now emboldened due to his new title.

Disputes had lately arisen between Miss Nightingale and some of the nurses in the Crimean hospitals. The situation had been embittered by rumours of religious dissensions, for, while the Crimean nurses were Roman Catholics, many of those at Scutari were suspected of a propensity towards the tenets of Protestantism. Miss Nightingale was by no means disturbed by these sectarian differences, but any suggestion that her supreme authority over all the nurses within the Army was enough to arouse her to fury, and it appeared that Sister Bridgman, the Reverend Mother in the Crimea, had ventured to call that authority into question. Sir John Hall thought that his opportunity had come, and strongly supported The Reverend Mother, or, as Miss Nightingale preferred to call her, the "Reverend Brickbat." There was a violent struggle and Miss Nightingale's rage was terrible. Dr. Hall, she declared, was doing his best to "root her out of the Crimea." She would bear it no longer; the War Office was attacking her falsely; there was only one thing to be done, Sidney Herbert must move for the production of papers in the House of Commons, so that the public might be able to judge between her and her enemies. Sidney Herbert, with great difficulty, calmed her down. Orders were immediately dispatched putting her supremacy beyond doubt, and the Reverend Mother Brickbat (Bridgman) withdrew from the scene. Sir John, however, was more tenacious. A few weeks later, Miss Nightingale and her nurses visited the Crimea for the last time, and the brilliant idea occurred to him that he could crush her by a very simple expedient. He could starve her into submission;

and he actually ordered that no rations of any kind should be supplied to her. He had already tried this plan with great effect upon an unfortunate medical man whose presence in the Crimea he had considered an intrusion, but he was now to learn that such tricks were thrown away upon Miss Nightingale. With extraordinary foresight, she had brought with her a great supply of food, and she succeeded in obtaining more at her own expense and by her own exertions. Thus for ten days, in that inhospitable country, she was able to feed herself and twenty-four nurses. Eventually the military authorities intervened in her favour, and Sir John had to confess that he was beaten.

It was not until July, 1856, four months after the Declaration of Peace, that Miss Nightingale left Scutari for England. Her reputation was now enormous, and the enthusiasm of the public was unbounded as she was mobbed everywhere she went. The Royal approbation was expressed by the gift of a brooch, accompanied by a private letter from Queen Victoria.

You are, I know, well aware [wrote Her Majesty] of the high sense I entertain of the Christian devotion which you have displayed during this great and bloody war, and I need hardly repeat to you how warm my admiration is for your services, which are fully equal to those of my dear and brave soldiers, whose sufferings you have had the privilege of alleviating in so merciful a manner. I am, however, anxious of marking my feelings in a manner which I trust will be agreeable to you, and therefore send you with this letter a brooch, the form and emblems of which commemorate your great and blessed work, and which I hope you will wear as a mark of the high approbation of your Sovereign. It will be a very great satisfaction to me to make the acquaintance of one who has set so bright an example to our sex. [11]

The brooch bore a St. George's cross and the royal cipher surrounded by diamonds. It had an inscription: "Blessed are the Merciful."

The name of Florence Nightingale lives in the memory of the world by virtue of the lurid and heroic adventure of the Crimea. Had she died, as she nearly did, upon her return to England, her reputation would hardly have been different. Her legend would have come down to us almost as we know it today of that gentle vision of female virtue which first took shape before the adoring eyes of the sick soldiers at Scutari. Yet, as a matter of fact, she lived for more than half a century after the Crimean War; and during the greater part of that long period all the energy and all the devotion of her extraordinary nature were working at their highest pitch. What she accomplished in those years of unknown labour could, indeed, hardly have been more glorious than her Crimean triumphs, but it was certainly more important in the development of nursing as an honoured and revered profession. The true history was far stranger even than the myth. In Miss Nightingale's own eyes, the adventure of the Crimea was a mere incident, scarcely more than a useful stepping-stone in her career. It was the pivotal moment with which she hoped to move the world, but other more momentous adventures lay ahead. For more than a generation she was to sit in secret, and her real life began at the very moment when, in the popular imagination, it had ended.

---

[11] Retrieved from
http://www.royalcollection.org.uk/egallery/exhibits.asp?exhibition=CRIMEA&exhibs=CRIMEA_06

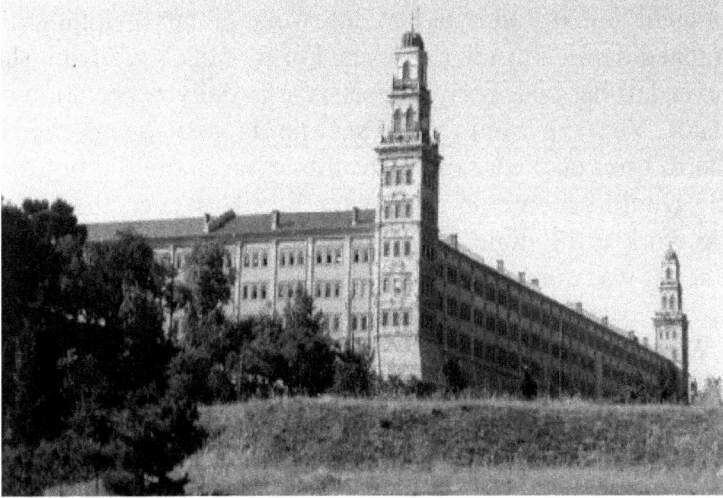

The old Barrack Hospital at Scutari still stands today. It is located on the Asian shore of the Bosphorus right opposite the peninsula of Istanbul.[12]

She arrived in England in a shattered state of health. The hardships and the ceaseless effort of the two years in Turkey had undermined her nervous system, her heart beat was irregular and she suffered constantly from fainting-spells. The doctors declared that one thing alone would save her, a complete and prolonged rest. However, that was also the one thing with which she would have nothing to do. She had never been in the habit of resting, so why should she begin now? After all, being famous would open great opportunities for her. No, she had work to do, and come what might, she would not rest on her laurels.

The doctors protested in vain, as did her family. A dedicated frenzy had seized upon her. She devoured books,

---

[12] Retrieved from http://www.florence-nightingale-avenging-angel.co.uk/scutari.htm.

dictated letters, and, in the intervals of her palpitations, cracked her health-related jokes. For months at a stretch she never left her bed. For years she was in daily expectation of death. Yet, she would not rest. The doctors assured her if she did not take care of her health, even if she did not die, she would become an invalid for life. However, there was the work to be done, and, as for rest, she would only rest when it was done.

Wherever she went, in London or in the country, in the hills of Derbyshire, or Embley, she was haunted by a ghost. It was the spectre of Scutari, the hideous vision of the organization of a military hospital. She would slay that phantom, or she would perish. The whole system of the Army Medical Department, the education of the Medical Officer, the regulations of hospital procedures were abominations. How could she rest while these things were as they were, knowing if war were to arise again, the like results would follow? And, even in peace and at home, what was the sanitary condition of the Army? The mortality in the barracks was, she found, nearly double the mortality in civilian life. "You might as well take 1100 men every year out upon Salisbury Plain and shoot them,"[13] she said. Scutari had given her knowledge; and it had given her power, too. Her enormous reputation was at her back, an incalculable force. Other work, other duties, might lie before her, but the most urgent, the most obvious of all was to look to the health of the Army.

One of her very first steps was to take advantage of the invitation which Queen Victoria had sent her to the Crimea, together with the commemorative brooch. Within a few

---

[13] Retrieved from
http://www.brainyquote.com/quotes/authors/f/florence_nightingal.html

weeks of her return, she visited the queen, and had several interviews both with the Queen and her husband. "She put before us," wrote the Prince in his diary, "all the defects of our present military hospital system and the reforms that are needed."[14]

But Miss Nightingale was not at the War Office, and for a very simple reason. She was a woman. Lord Panmure, however, was, and it was upon Lord Panmure that the issue of Miss Nightingale's efforts for reform depended. He had come into office in the middle of the Sebastopol campaign of the Crimean War, and had felt himself very well fitted for the position, since he had acquired in former days an inside knowledge of the Army as a captain in the cavalry. It was this inside knowledge which had enabled him to inform Miss Nightingale with such authority that "the British soldier was not a remitting animal." Though he did not dislike her, he saw her as a nuisance.

At the first meeting, he brought a phalanx of professional conservatism, the stubborn supporters of the out-of-date, the worshippers and the victims of War Office routine. Among these it was only natural that Dr. Andrew Smith, the head of the Army Medical Department, should have been pre-eminent. The same Dr. Andrew Smith, who had assured Miss Nightingale before she left England that "nothing was wanted at Scutari."[15] Such were her opponents, but she, too, was not without allies. She had gained the ear of Royalty, which was something she used frequently to gain the ear of the public. She had a host of

---

[14]Retrieved from
http://www.history1800s.about.com/od/majorfigures/p/fnightingale01.htm
[15] Retrieved from http://www.florence-nightingale-avenging-angel.co.uk/scutari.htm

admirers and friends, to say nothing of her personal qualities - her knowledge, her tenacity, her tact, and she also belonged to the highest circle of society. She moved naturally among the privileged classes. What kind of attention would such persons have paid to some middle-class woman with whom they were not acquainted, and who possessed great experience of army nursing and had determined views about hospital reform? They would have politely ignored her, but it was impossible to ignore Florence Nightingale. When she spoke, they were obliged to listen, and, when they had once begun to do that, she was capable of weaving a spell that seemed to captivate them. She supported her weightiest minutes with familiar witty little notes. These men were no match for this small, determined lady.

Of Miss Nightingale's friends, the most important was Sidney Herbert. He was a man of enviable gifts. Well born, handsome, rich, the master of Wilton, one of the greatest country-houses in all of England. He was clothed with the glamour of a historic past, which is the peculiar glory of the out-dated but ever prevalent English class system, and he possessed, besides all these advantages, so charming, so lively, so gentle, so serene a disposition that no one who had once come near him could ever be his enemy.

His career would certainly have been very different if he had never known Florence Nightingale. The alliance between them, which had begun with her appointment to Scutari, which had grown closer and closer while the war lasted, developed, after her return, into one of the most extraordinary of friendships. It was the friendship of a man and a woman intimately bound together by their devotion to a public cause and mutual affection. In all likelihood, it was an intensely intimate relationship. For years, Sidney

Herbert saw Miss Nightingale almost daily, for long hours together, corresponding with her incessantly when they were apart, but the wagging tongues of scandal were, for the most part, silent. In fact, one of Miss Nightingale's most devoted admirers was Herbert's wife. But what made the connection still more remarkable was the way in which the parts that were played in it were divided between the two. Generally, at this time in history, it was the man who acted, decided, and achieved, while it was the woman who encouraged, applauded, and inspired. In this case, these roles were reversed; the qualities of pliancy and sympathy fell to the man, those of command and initiative, to the woman. There was one thing only which Miss Nightingale lacked in her equipment for public life, she lacked and could never get the public power and authority which belong to the successful politician. That power and authority Sidney Herbert possessed. It was through this man that Florence worked her will. She took hold of him, taught him, shaped him, absorbed him, dominated him to the extreme. He did not resist, as his natural inclination lay along the same path as hers. Her strong personality swept him forward at her own fierce pace and with her own relentless dedication. Although a woman of deep substance, Florence was also a woman of immense feminine charms who was not above using those charms to achieve her goals.

Besides Sidney Herbert, Florence had other friends who, in a more restricted sphere, were hardly less essential to her. If, in her condition of bodily collapse, she were to accomplish what she was determined to achieve, the attentions and the services of others would be absolutely indispensable. Helpers and servers she must have; and accordingly there was soon formed about her a little group of devoted disciples upon whose affections and energies she could implicitly rely. Devoted, indeed, these disciples were, because she was an exacting task-master.

Yet, she never asked of others that which she, herself, would not do. So the little band, bound body and soul in strange servitude to a woman as well as a cause, laboured on ungrudgingly. Among the most faithful was her "Aunt Mai," her father's sister, who from the earliest days had stood beside her, who had helped her to escape from the humdrum of family life. She had been with her at Scutari, and watched over her with infinite care in all the movements and uncertainties which her state of health involved. Another constant attendant was her brother-in-law, Sir Harry Verney, whom she found particularly valuable in parliamentary affairs. Arthur Clough, the poet, also a connection by marriage, she used in other ways.

As time went on, her "Cabinet," as she called it, grew larger. Officials with whom she had contact and those who sympathized with her goals, were pressed into service as a result of her indomitable personality, and old friends of the Crimean days gathered round her constantly. Among these the most indefatigable was Dr. Sutherland, a sanitary expert, who for more than thirty years acted as her confidential private secretary, and surrendered to her purposes literally the whole of his life.

The first great measure, which, supported as it was by the Queen, the Cabinet, and the united opinion of the country, was the appointment of a Royal Commission to report upon the health of the Army. The question of the composition of the Commission then immediately arose, and it was over this matter that a first face-to-face encounter between Lord Panmure and Miss Nightingale took place. They met, and

Miss Nightingale was victorious; Sidney Herbert was appointed Chairman, and in the end the only member of the commission opposed to her views was Dr. Andrew Smith. During the process, Miss Nightingale made an important discovery. She found that these people who wanted to keep things as they were feared an appeal to public opinion. The faintest hint of such a terrible eventuality made their hearts dissolve within them. Miss Nightingale held the fearful threat in reserve at all times, as she knew they feared that she would speak out and that she would publish the truth to the whole world, and let the whole world judge for themselves. With supreme skill, she held this sword poised above the heads of those who refused to support progressive measures in healthcare.

Was the commission to be efficiently armed with the right of full and unfettered inquiry or was it to be a polite official contrivance for exonerating Dr. Andrew Smith and the others who refused to look after the needs of the country's soldiers? The War Office phalanx closed its ranks, and fought tooth and nail, but it was defeated, as a result of the sheer will of one woman, Florence Nightingale.

Lord Panmure cowered into submission once more, as he had immediately hurried to the Queen to obtain her consent, and only then, when Queen Victoria's initials had been irrevocably affixed to the fatal document, did he dare to tell Dr. Andrew Smith what he had done. The Commission met, and another immense load fell upon Miss Nightingale's shoulders. Today she would, of course, have been a member of the Commission herself, but at that time, the idea of a woman appearing in such a capacity was unheard of, and no one even suggested the possibility of Miss Nightingale's doing so. The result was that she was obliged to remain behind the scenes throughout, to coach Sidney Herbert in private at every important juncture, and to convey to him and to her other friends upon the Commission the vast reservoir of her expert knowledge. She was only allowed to give evidence in written form. The Commission's Report, embodying almost word for word the suggestions of Miss Nightingale, was drawn up by Sidney Herbert. Only one question remained to be answered—would anything, after all, be done? Or would the Royal Commission, like so many other Royal Commissions before and since, achieve nothing but the concoction of a very fat pack of papers that would gather dust.

And so the last and the deadliest struggle began. Six months had been spent in coercing Lord Panmure into granting the Commission effective powers. Six more months were occupied by the work of the Commission, and now yet another six were to pass in extorting from him the means whereby the recommendations of the Commission might be actually carried out. But, in the end, the thing was done. Miss Nightingale seemed indeed, during these months, to be upon the very brink of death. Accompanied by the faithful Aunt Mai, she moved from place to place in what appeared to be a last desperate effort to find health somewhere; but she carried on with that which made health impossible, as her desire for work could scarcely be distinguished from mania. At one moment she was writing a "last letter" to Sidney Herbert. At the next she was offering nursing services as far away as India. Yet, through it all, her obsessive nature never diminished, as it seemed the only thing that mattered to her was seeing that those in need were justly served.

Her wits began to turn, and there was no holding her. She worked like a slave driven by a demanding overseer. She began to believe, as she had begun to believe at Scutari, that none of her fellow-workers had their hearts in the business, because if they had, why did they not work as she did? She could only see slackness and stupidity around her. The fate of the vital recommendation in the Commission's Report, the appointment of four Sub-Commissions charged with the duty of determining upon the details of the proposed reforms and of putting them into execution, still hung in the balance. However, through determination and an indomitable will Florence eventually got her way.

Events turned dramatically when Sidney Herbert became Secretary of State for War. The next two and a half years (1859–61) saw the introduction of the whole system of reforms for which Miss Nightingale had been struggling so fiercely, reforms which make Sidney Herbert's tenure of power at the War Office an important epoch in the history of the British Army. The four Sub-Commissions, firmly established under the immediate control of the Minister, and urged forward by the relentless perseverance of Miss Nightingale, set to work with a will. The barracks and the hospitals were remodelled. They were properly ventilated and warmed and lighted for the first time. They were given a water supply which actually supplied water, and in the kitchens, strange to say, it was possible to cook. Then the great question of the quartermaster, that portentous functionary whose powers and whose lack of powers had weighed like a nightmare upon Scutari, was taken in hand, and new regulations were laid down, accurately defining his responsibilities and his duties. One Sub-Commission reorganized the medical statistics of the Army. Another established an Army Medical School. Finally the Army Medical Department itself was completely reorganized, an administrative code was drawn up and the great and novel principle was established that it was as much a part of the duty of the authorities to look after the soldier's health as to look after his sickness. Besides this, it was at last officially admitted that the soldier had a moral and intellectual side. Coffee-rooms and reading-rooms, gymnasiums and workshops were instituted. A new era did in truth appear to have begun. Already by 1861 the mortality in the Army had decreased by one half since the days of the Crimea. It was no wonder that even vaster possibilities began now to open before Miss Nightingale. One thing was still needed to complete and to assure her triumphs. The Army Medical Department was indeed reorganized, but the War Office itself was still untouched. If she could remould that nearer to her heart's desire, that indeed would be a victory. Until that final act was accomplished, how could she be certain that all the rest of her achievements might not, by some capricious whim, be abrogated by someone who was a puppet to the War Office?

Her concerns were bolstered when Sidney Herbert had consented to undertake the reform of the War Office. He had sallied forth into that tropical jungle of festooned obstructionism, of inter-twisted irresponsibility, of crouching prejudices, of abuses grown stiff and rigid with antiquity, which for so many years to come would lure reforming ministers to their doom.

To quote Florence, "the War Office is a very slow office, an enormously expensive office, and one in which the Minister's intentions can be entirely negated by all his sub-departments, and those of each of the sub-departments by every other department."[16]

---

[16] Retrieved from
http://www.brainyquote.com/quotes/authors/f/florence_nightingal.html

At the first rumour of a change, the old phalanx of reaction was bristling with its accustomed spears. At its head stood no longer Dr. Andrew Smith, who, some time since, had the good grace to succumb to old age, but a yet more formidable figure, the permanent Under-Secretary himself, Sir Benjamin Hawes, a man remarkable even among civil servants for adroitness in baffling inconvenient inquiries, resourceful in raising false issues, and, in short, a consummate command of all the arts of officially fighting the encroachment of reformers. "Our scheme will probably result in Ben Hawes's resignation," Miss Nightingale said; "and that is another of its advantages."[17]

Ben Hawes himself, however, did not quite see it in that light. He set himself to resist the wishes of the Minister by every means in his power. The struggle was long and desperate; and, as it proceeded, it gradually became evident to Miss Nightingale that something was wrong with Sidney Herbert. What was it? His health, never very strong, was, he said, in danger of collapsing under the strain of his work. But, after all, what is illness, when there is a War Office to be reorganized? Then he began to talk of retiring altogether from public life. The doctors were consulted, and declared that, above all things, rest was necessary. This suggestion alarmed Florence. Was it possible that, at the last moment, the crowning wreath of victory was to be snatched from her grasp? She was not to be put aside by doctors; they were talking nonsense; the necessary thing was not rest but the reform of the War Office, and, she knew very well from her own case what one could do even when one was on the point of death. She expostulated

---

[17] Retrieved from
http://www.history1800s.about.com/od/majorfigures/p/fnightingale01.htm

vehemently and passionately that with the goal so near, he could not rest now.

Typically, Sidney Herbert could not resist Miss Nightingale. A compromise was arranged. Very reluctantly, he exchanged the turmoil of the House of Commons for the dignity of the House of Lords, and he remained at the War Office. She was delighted. "One fight more, the best and the last,"[18] she said.

For several more months the fight did indeed go on, but the strain upon Herbert was greater even than Florence perhaps realized. His health grew worse. He was attacked by fainting-fits, and there were some days when he could only just keep himself going by gulps of brandy. Miss Nightingale spurred him forward with her encouragements and her admonitions, her zeal and her example. However, at last his spirit began to sink as well as his body. He could no longer hope to implement the reforms needed. He had failed. The dreadful moment came when the truth was forced upon him. He would never be able to reform the War Office. Yet, the real dread was having to face Florence and tell her that he was a failure, a beaten man.

How ironic that the broach given her by Queen Victoria was engraved with the words, "blessed are the merciful," because she showed no mercy in attacking her friend, Sidney Herbert. Turning to him in fury when he said he was a beaten man, she let out a torrent of emotion. "Beaten! Can't you see that you've simply thrown away the game? And with all the winning cards in your hands! And so noble a game! Sidney Herbert beaten! And beaten by

---

[18] Retrieved from
http://www.brainyquote.com/quotes/authors/f/florence_nightingal.html

Ben Hawes! It is a worse disgrace than the hospitals at Scutari."

He dragged himself away from her, dragged himself to a Spa, hoping vainly for a return of health, and then, despairing, back again to England, to Wilton, to the majestic house standing there resplendent in the summer sunshine, offering a modicum of solace from the brow-beating he had suffered at the hands of his beloved Florence. He returned to Wilton and lay in a near comatose state. After having received the Eucharist, he had become perfectly calm. Then, almost unconscious, his lips were seen to be moving. Those about him bent down and heard his final words, "Poor Florence! Poor Florence!" as he embraced the peace only offered him in death.[19]

If Miss Nightingale had been less ruthless, Sidney Herbert may not have perished when he did. The force that created was also the force that destroyed. It was her inner demons that were responsible for her reprehensible behaviour. When the fatal news reached her, she was overcome by agony. In the revulsion of her feelings, she began to worship the dead man's memory. The faithful Aunt Mai did not, to be sure, die; no, she did something almost worse: she left Florence Nightingale. She was growing old, and she felt that she had closer and more imperative duties with her own family. Her niece could hardly forgive her. She poured out, in one of her enormous letters, a passionate diatribe upon the faithlessness, the lack of sympathy, the stupidity, the ineptitude of women. Her doctrines had taken no hold among them. They were nothing but servile minions worshipping at the feet of men.

[19] Bostridge,M. (2008) *Florence Nightingale. The Woman and Her Legend.* New York, New York, Viking Press.

She felt deserted in her hour of deepest need. With Sidney gone, she had nothing but her work, and her work was her salvation.

Sidney Herbert's death finally put an end to Miss Nightingale's dream of a reformed War Office. Succeeding Secretaries of State managed between them to undo a good deal of what had been accomplished, but they could not undo it all, and for ten years more (1862–72) Miss Nightingale remained a potent influence at the War Office. After that, her direct connection with the army came to an end, and her energies began to turn more and more completely towards more general objects. Her work on hospital reform assumed enormous proportions. She was able to improve the conditions in infirmaries and workhouses. She set up a training school for nurses and began work to improve medical conditions in colonial India. Her tentacles reached into the India Office and succeeded in establishing such a hold there that the newly appointed Viceroy of India, before he left England, paid a courtesy call on her to ask for advice.

After much hesitation, she settled down in a small house on South Street in London, where she remained for the rest of her life. That life was a very long one, as she lived until she was 91.. Her ill-health gradually diminished, the crises of extreme danger became less frequent, and at last, altogether ceased. She remained an invalid, but an invalid of a curious character, an invalid who was too weak to walk downstairs and who worked far harder than most Cabinet Ministers. Her illness, whatever it may have been, was certainly not inconvenient. It involved much seclusion. Butt lying on her sofa in a little upper room on South Street, she combined the intense vitality of a dominating woman of the world with the mysterious and romantic quality of a myth. She was a legend in her lifetime, and she knew it.

She tasted the joys of immense power and wide-spread fame. Great statesmen and renowned generals were obliged to beg for audiences. Admirers from foreign countries found that they must see her at her own time, or not at all; and the ordinary mortal had no hope of ever getting beyond the downstairs sitting-room past her devoted doctor, John Sutherland, who rarely left her alone. Downstairs he sat, transacting business, answering correspondence, interviewing callers, and exchanging innumerable notes for Florence with other powerful figures. Sometimes word came down that Miss Nightingale was just well enough to see one of her visitors. The fortunate man was led up, was ushered, trembling, into the shaded chamber, and, of course, could never afterwards forget the interview. Very rarely, indeed, once or twice a year, perhaps, but nobody could be quite certain, in deadly secrecy, Miss Nightingale went out for a drive in the park. Unrecognized, the living legend flitted for a moment before the common gaze. Precaution was necessary; for there were times when, at some public function, the rumour of her presence was spread and ladies would vehemently ask, "let me touch your shawl," or "let me stroke your arm." This strange adoration never ceased in her lifetime.

Those in power still feared her influence as she would remind some timid minister, or some un-persuadable bureaucrat, sitting in audience with her in the little upper room, that she was something more than a mere sick woman, that she had only to go to the window and wave her handkerchief, and dreadful things would follow. The myth was almost reality as she was obstinate, portentous and impalpable to the last.

With statesmen and officials at her beck and call, with her hands on a hundred strings, with mighty worshippers at her feet, with foreign governments agog for her counsel, building hospitals and training nurses, she still felt there were more worlds to conquer.

When old age actually came, something curious happened. Destiny, having waited very patiently, played a queer trick on Miss Nightingale. The benevolence and public spirit had only been equalled by her use of bitterness toward those who stood in her way. The sarcastic years brought the proud woman her punishment, because she was not to die as she had lived. The sting was to be taken out of her. She was to be made soft and reduced to compliance and complacency. The change came gradually, but at last it was unmistakable. The terrible commander who had driven Sidney Herbert to his death, and struck fear into the hearts of many, now accepted small compliments with gratitude, and indulged in sentimental friendships with young girls. The author of the renowned and still revered *Notes on Nursing*, that classical compendium of nursing knowledge, drawn up with the detailed acrimony and vindictive relish, spent long hours in composing sympathetic addresses to individuals whom she pitied and often wept over. And, at the same time there appeared a corresponding alteration in her physical mould. The thin, angular woman, with her haughty eye and her acrid mouth had vanished, and in her place was the rounded bulky form of a rotund old lady, smiling all day long. Then something else became visible. The brain which had been steeled at Scutari was indeed, literally, growing soft. Senility descended on her. Towards the end, consciousness itself grew lost in a haze, and melted into nothingness. It was just then, three years before her death, when she was eighty-seven years old (1907), that those in authority thought that the opportune moment had come for bestowing a public honour on Florence Nightingale. She was offered the Order of Merit for a life of selfless devotion to the care of the sick. Miss Nightingale's representatives accepted the honour, and her name, after a lapse of many years, once more appeared in the press. The medal was brought to her bedside, where she fondled it and smiled. The lady who was intense, driven and often intolerable to deal with, but admirable in her achievements, had, no doubt, mellowed with age. In tribute, when she died, several of her devotees stood outside her home carrying lamps in memory of the "lady with a lamp," who prowled the wards of Scutari to bring solace to those who suffered.

There are conflicting reports of her final words, but being incurable romantics, we prefer to believe the account that said they were, "my dear Sidney, I am sorry."[20]

---

[20] Retrieved from
http://www.brainyquote.com/quotes/authors/f/florence_nightingal.html

Statue of Florence Nightingale in Waterloo Place, London, UK[21]

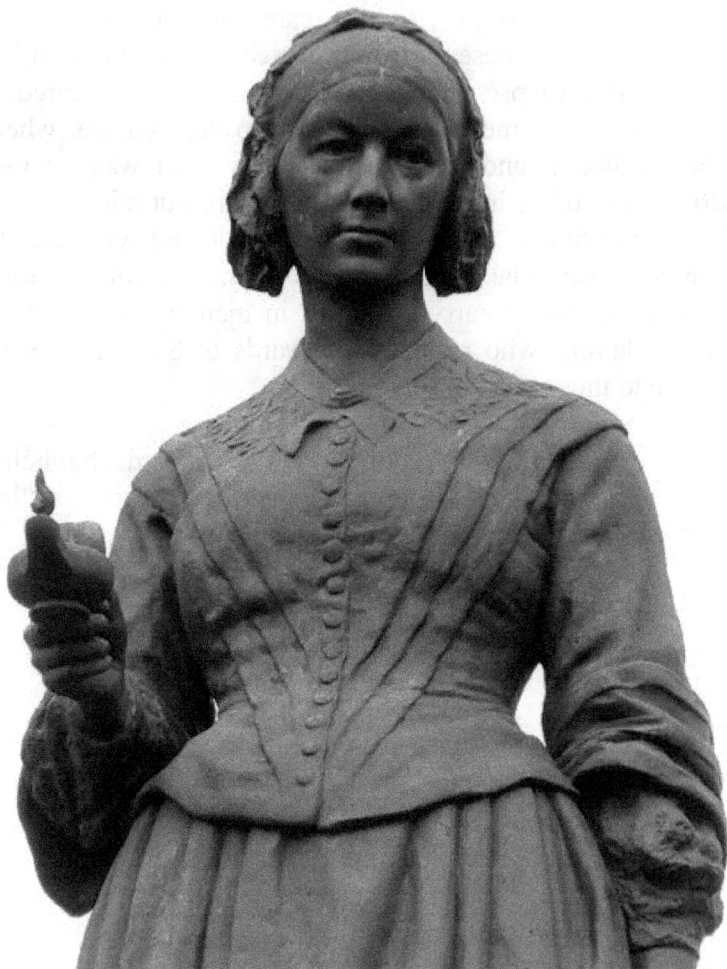

Always revered as "The Lady with a Lamp,"
this statue was erected in her memory in 1912.

---

[21] Retrieved from
wikimedia.org/wiki/File:Statue_to_Florence_Nightingale,_Waterloo_ .
Place,_London_W1_-_geograph.org.uk_-_894231.jpg

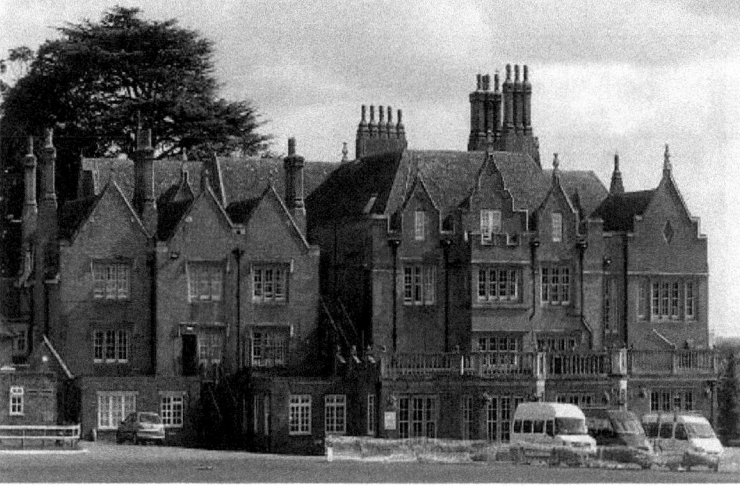

Embley Park, Now a School, Was One of the Many Family Homes Of Florence's Father, William Nightingale[22]

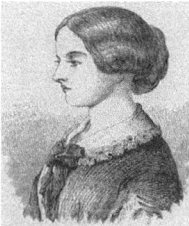

Portrait Of
Florence
Nightingale
(Circa 1851)[24]

NIGHTINGALE NURSE'S PLEDGE[23]

I solemnly pledge myself before God and in the presence of this assembly, to pass my life in purity and to practice my profession faithfully. I will abstain from whatever is deleterious and mischievous, and will not take or knowingly administer any harmful drug. I will do all in my power to maintain and elevate the standard of my profession, and will hold in confidence all personal matters committed to my keeping and all family affairs coming to my knowledge in the practice of my calling. With loyalty will I endeavour to aid the physician, in his work, and devote myself to the welfare of those committed to my care.

---

[22] Retrieved from http://en.wikipedia.org/wiki/Florence_Nightingale
[23] Retrieved from http://www.carenurse.com/creeds/nightingale.html
[24] Retrieved from http://en.wikipedia.org/wiki/Florence_Nightingale

Nightingale Receiving the Wounded at Scutari by Jerry Barrett 1906[25]

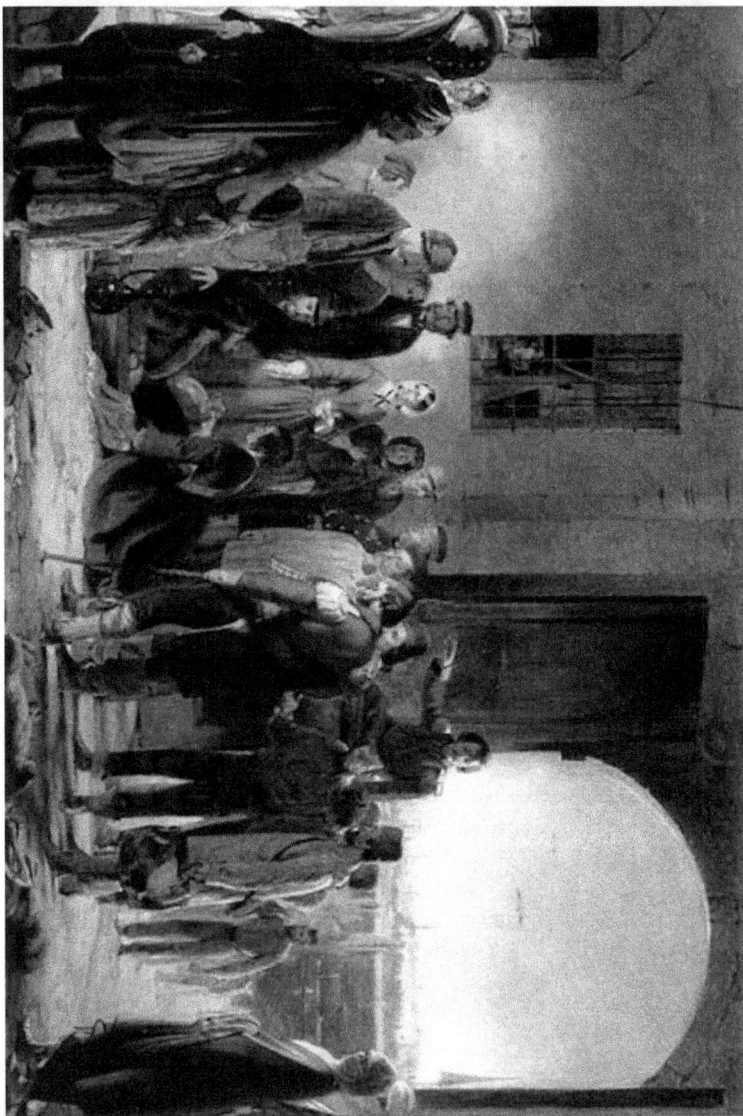

[25] Retrieved from
http://www.nationalportraitgallery/London/lithographs.uk

Famous Florence Nightingale Quotes[26]

How very little can be done under the spirit of fear.

I attribute my success to this - I never gave or took any excuse.

I have lived and slept in the same bed with English countesses and Prussian farm women... no woman has excited passions among women more than I have.

I think one's feelings waste themselves in words; they ought all to be distilled into actions which bring results.

It may seem a strange principle to enunciate as the very first requirement in a hospital that it should do the sick no harm.

So never lose an opportunity of urging a practical beginning, however small, for it is wonderful how often in such matters the mustard-seed germinates and roots itself.

The world is put back by the death of every one who has to sacrifice the development of his or her peculiar gifts to conventionality.

Were there none who were discontented with what they have, the world would never reach anything better.

You ask me why I do not write something.... I think one's feelings waste themselves in words, they ought all to be

[26] Retrieved fromhttp://www.brainyquote.com/quotes/authors/f/florence_nightingale.html

distilled into actions and into actions which bring results.

I ask no more of anyone than I ask of myself

CHAPTER 5
GEORGINA FANE POPE
A WOMAN OF DEEP COMPASION
FOR THOSE WHO NEEDED IT MOST

Born in Charlottetown, Prince Edward Island, Georgina Pope was the daughter of William Pope, a "Father of Canadian Confederation." A product of Prince Edward Island gentility, Georgina, doubtless, could have had a comfortable marriage and become an island socialite as did all her other female relatives. Instead, like Florence Nightingale, she turned her back on the conventional and expected and to pursue a career in nursing by attending the leading American school of nursing at Bellevue in New York City. She worked in New York for awhile, before returning to Canada to seek a position as a nurse with the troops departing for South Africa to fight in the Boar War.

Pope was the first permanent member of the Canadian Army Nursing Service, a distinction that she was proud of all her life. Along with four other nurses, she accompanied Canada's first military contingent to South Africa and was given the honorary rank of lieutenant. For five grueling months after their arrival, the first group, with Georgina Pope as the senior nurse, served at British hospitals and aid stations just north of Cape Town, South Africa. Then, Nurse Pope, along with another nurse proceeded north to Kroonstadt, where, despite shortages of food and medical supplies, they took charge of the military hospital, successfully caring for 230 sufferers of enteric fever and other patients who had various other maladies. Shortly afterward, she returned home but in January 1902, Pope returned to South Africa a second time as senior nurse in charge of a second group of eight Canadian nurses. Three other nurses among them were returning for a second tour of duty. They served at a hospital in Natal until the end of the war.[27]

In 1903, Pope was recognized for her service in the field of nursing, and was the first Canadian to be awarded the Royal Red Cross by Queen Victoria.[28] In 1906, Nurse Pope began work as a member of the permanent Canadian Army Medical Corps at the Garrison Hospital in Halifax. Two years later, she attained the position of matron, the first in the history of the Canadian Army Medical Corps. Nurse Pope went overseas again in 1917 (World War I) and served in the U.K. and then in France at the front line hospitals.

Georgia oversaw recruitment for many years and her main duties werein hospital administration. A visible mark of Georgina's presence was her decision to change the nursing sisters' uniforms from khaki colour to navy blue. She also added an insignia in the shape of a maple leaf with a crown placed over the word Canada.

For a period of many years, just like Florence Nightingale, Georgina suffered poor health. Yet, even poor health did not keep her from serving in World War I, when at the age of 55, she volunteered for duty on the Western Front. She was near many fierce battles, including Ypres. Succumbing to another bout of illness, which may have included shell-shock , she was sent home to Canada in August 1918. Retiring, Georgina lived in her hometown of Charlottetown, Prince Edward Island until she died on June 6, 1938. She was 76 years old.

---

[27]Retrieved from.http://www.warmuseum.ca/cwm/exhibitions/boer/georginapope_e.shtml

[28] Retrieved from http://www.liberalsenateforum.ca/In-The-Senate/Statement/1656

Matron-in-Chief Georgina Fane Pope was buried in the Charlottetown Roman Catholic Cemetery with full military honors. Again, like Florence Nightingale, she did not marry or have any children, as her work was her life.[29]

In 2006, the Valiants Memorial on Confederation Square was dedicated in Ottawa, Ontario. It consists of 14 busts and statues of Canadian military heroes. There are two women honoured, one of them is Georgina Fane Pope.

Although we tend to make heroes out of those who go into battle and overcome great odds, the simple dedication of women like Georgina Fane Pope should make us all realize that heroes do not have to go into battle to receive our adulation. It is often those who serve quietly who also deserve recognition. Nurses like Georgina Fane Pope braved the horrors of war to reach out with the hand of compassion to those who were wounded, maimed and broken on the fields of horror.

How fitting that among all the heroes displayed in bronze at the Valiants Memorial is one who never fired a shot in anger at anyone, but simply made sure that those who suffered physical and mental anguish had the best medical care possible. Although not a lady with a lamp, Georgina Fane Pope, was a woman with a kind heart who always strived to provide the best care possible for her patients.

Although not as famous as Lieutenant Colonel John McCrae's immortal *"In Flanders Fields"*, many Canadians found the below Canadian nurses' ballad almost as endearing and emotional.

---

[29] Retrieved from http://susanna-mcleod.suite101.com/georgina-fane-pope-first-matron-of-canadian-army-nursing-corps-a288606

Nursing Sisters' Theme Song[30]

In my sweet little Alice Blue gown,
When I first came to Birmingham town.
I had had a bad trip, in a nasty old ship
And the cold in my billet, just gave me the pip.
We came out to nurse our own troops,
But were greeted with measles and whoops.
Now I'll be a granny, and sit on my fanny,
And keep warm with turpentine stupes.

In my sweet little Alice Blue gown,
When I return to my home town
They will bring out the band, give the girls a big hand,
Being a nurse in the force, I'll be quite renowned.
And I'll never forget all the fun,
That I had, since I joined Number One
I was happy and gay, to have served with MacRae
In my sweet little Alice Blue gown.

Although she is not as renowned as Florence Nightingale, Pope is considered the Canadian equivalent. During her lifetime, she was highly venerated and admired. In 1918, a returning war veteran said of her, "she was an angel of mercy in the field hospital where so many of us lay broken

---

[30] Retrieved from
http://www.oshawaremembers.wordpress.com/2008/11/28/story-fifty-eight-canadian-nurses-angels-of-mercy/

in body and spirit. She was a woman of deep compassion for those who needed it most."[31]

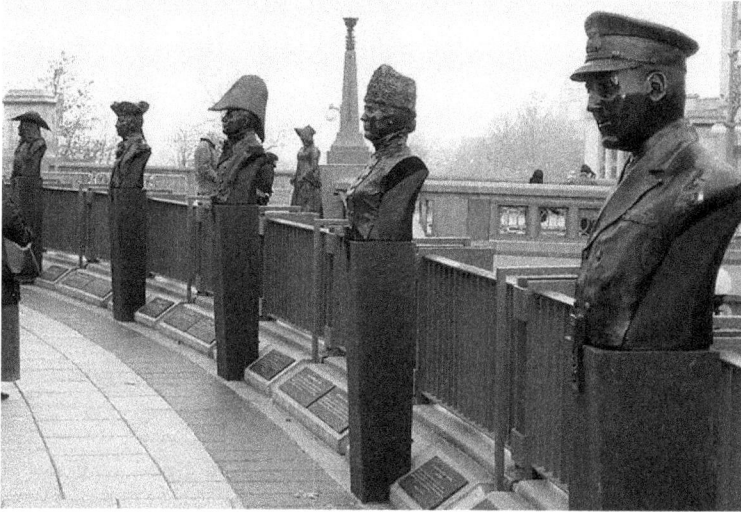

Valiants Memorial[32]

A bronze bust of Pope (2nd from right) has been erected to commemorate her contribution to Canadian military history as part of the Valiants Memorial in Confederation Square in downtown Ottawa. This national monument was unveiled on November 5, 2006, as part of Veterans' Week. The memorial honours 14 Canadians for their service during five separate wars.

The inscription on the wall below the monument in Confederation Square captures the spirit of the memorial: "No day shall ever erase you from the memory of time."[33]

---

[31] Retrieved from http://www.quotesfromthegreatwar.ca
[32] Retrieved from
http://www.en.wikipedia.org/wiki/Valiants_Memorial

Encapsulated History Of Georgina Fane Pope

Birth:
1 January 1862 in Charlottetown, Prince Edward Island, Canada

Death:
6 June 1938 in Charlottetown, Prince Edward Island, Canada

Education:
School of Nursing, Belleview Hospital, New York City, New York, USA

Career
of
Georgina Fane Pope
In Abbreviated Form

- After nursing school in New York City, Georgina Fane Pope began her nursing career in the United States, where she worked in civic hospitals.
- She came back to Canada to volunteer as a nurse to go overseas with the troops leaving for the South African War in late 1899.
- Georgina Fane Pope was the senior nursing sister of the four nurses who went with the first Canadian troops to South Africa. Four more nurses followed. The nurses were given the rank, pay and benefits of lieutenant.
- For five months Georgina Fane Pope worked at British hospitals just north of Cape Town.

---

[33] Retrieved from http://www.canadascapital.gc.ca/places-to-visit/public-art/valiants-memorial

- Georgina Fane Pope then went to Kroonstadt, where she and another nursing sister took charge of the military hospital, caring for more than 200 patients, most with enteric fever.
- At the end of 1900, Georgina Fane Pope returned to Canada and was put on reserve status.
- In 1901, the Canadian Army Nursing Service was made official, and Georgina Fane Pope was one of its seven members.
- In 1902, Georgina Fane Pope went back to South Africa. She served in a hospital in Natal until the end of the South African War.
- In 1903, Georgina Fane Pope was awarded the Royal Red Cross by Queen Victoria for conspicuous service in the field. She was the first Canadian to receive the award.
- In 1906, Georgina Fane Pope became a member of the new permanent Canadian Army Medical Corps and worked at the Garrison military hospital in Halifax, Nova Scotia. She was responsible for a handful of permanent staff and up to 80 reservists by 1914.
- In 1908, she was appointed Nursing Matron, the first in the Canadian Army Medical Corps.
- In 1917, Georgina Fane Pope again went overseas, this time to serve in England and France in World War I. She was sent back to Canada in 1918, suffering from health problems, including shell shock.
- She retired to Prince Edward Island.
- When Georgina Fane Pope died in 1938, she was given a full military funeral.

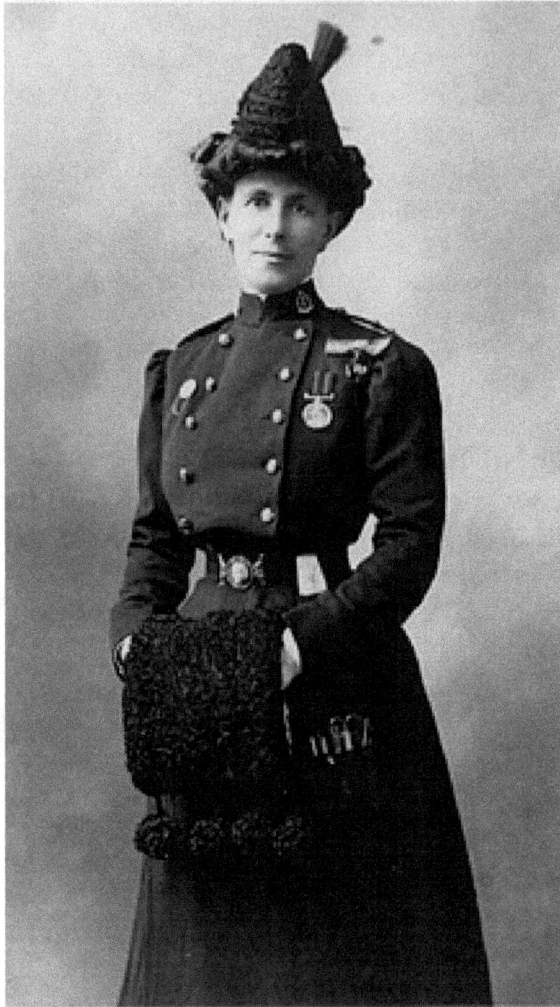

Georgia Fane Pope in South Africa
(The Boar War 1899-1902)[34]

---

[34] Retrieved from
www.warmuseum.ca/cwm/exhibitions/boer/georginapope_e.shtml

CHAPTER 6
MARY MEAGRE SOUTHCOTT
THE FLORENCE NIGHTINGALE OF
NEWFOUNDLAND

Mary Meager Southcott was born in St. John's, Newfoundland on 21 September 1862 and is considered one of the foremost nursing pioneers in Canada. She completed her basic nursing program and certificate in midwifery from the London Hospital Training School in England. However, she was the oldest student at school. How she wound up there at the age of 37, is itself, an interesting story that involves a romantic interlude.

Botany was a hobby for Mary, and through that hobby she also developed an interest in water colours, as she enjoyed painting the flora of the countryside. A local minister, Reverend Arthur Waghrone, showed an interest in her paintings, and they developed a romantic attachment. In 1888, they announced their engagement. However within a year the engagement was cancelled due to what Reverend Waghrone termed irreversible financial loses on his part. Apparently, Mary was devastated by the whole affair and went through many years of emotional pain as a result. Financially independent through an inheritance, in 1899 Southcott went to nursing school in London, where she was trained by a Florence Nightingale protégé.

On 1 March 1901, she received her graduation certificate and was commended for her superior skills. She then went on to study midwifery, and upon return to St. John's she was appointed Superintendent of Nurses at St. Johns in 1903. Like Florence Nightingale, she was strong-willed, and felt that nurses should be accorded great respect for their knowledge. She established the first school of nursing in Newfoundland, which was modelled on the Nightingale system, and she formed the Association of Registered Nurses of Newfoundland and Labrador. When she started her career, she was paid the princely sum of $480 a year ($12,000 in 2011 Canadian dollars).

The regulations for admission reflected Southcott's dedication to attracting superior applicants as they had to be between the age of 21 and 30 years, unmarried, of average height, in good health, and have a good common school education, or pass the entrance examination provided by Southcott. Since she followed the Nightingale system, there was a strict secular approach to the training. However, religion did play a significant
role in Mary Southcott's life as she was a devout member of the Church of England, and it actually may have been a contributing factor to a feud that developed between her and Dr. Lawrence Keegan, the Medical Superintendent at the General Hospital, who was Roman Catholic. What follows is a paraphrased account of the turmoil as stated by Linda White in her 1994 article *Who's in Charge Here? The General Hospital School of Nursing, St John's, Newfoundland* (White, 1994).[35]

At the core of the Nightingale plan was the absolute supremacy of the Superintendent of Nurses over all nurses and midwives. Thus, developed a schism between Southcott and Keegan. As Superintendent of the General Hospital, Keegan thought that the Nightingale concept was outmoded, and that it was he who should have final say in all matters concerning nurses.

---

[35] White, L. (1994). *Who's in Charge Here? The General Hospital School of Nursing, St John's, Newfoundland* 1903-1930.CBMH/BCHM /Volume11:1993, pp.91-118.

In 1914, Keegan was closely connected to the Conservative party and went over Southcott's head to make two graduate nurse appointments based on patronage (their father's were strong supporters of the Conservative party). Additionally, Keegan was accused of misappropriating food and hospital supplies for his personal use by an opposition member in Parliament. Since the Conservative party had a majority, no inquiry was ever conducted.

Meanwhile, in order to draw attention away from the accusations, Keegan publicly stated that he was being undermined in the effective running of the hospital by Southcott and her nurses. He insisted that he had the right to make nurses appointments, not Southcott.

All this a rancour had developed over a period of time when Keegan was constantly trying to usurp Southcott's authority. The conflict can be traced back as far as 1912 when Southcott had promised Elizabeth Redmond the position of matron of the newly built King Edward VII Home for Nurses. Keegan insisted that the position go to another nurse, Annie Cashin. Keegan told Southcott that the government was proposing a new position, Assistant Superintendent of Nurses, and that Redmond deserved that position. Southcott agreed. Yet, when the new position was created, Keegan arranged with the government to have someone else appointed. Two years later, on 17 March 1914, when that person resigned, Southcott was determined to regain her right of assigning staff and appointed Redmond to the post immediately. Southcott felt that after so many years of service, mostly on night duty, Redmond deserved the position. A few days later, Keegan encountered Redmond and Southcott on a ward with Bertha Forsey, the sister in charge. Keegan asked Redmond in what capacity she was working on the ward. She responded that she was the Assistant Superintendent of Nurses. Enraged, Keegan ordered her off the ward. In solidarity, Southcott and Forsey also left the ward. Later that night and during the early hours of the next morning, the sisters and staff nurses gathered in the nurses' residence to talk over the day's events and to discuss what action they would take in response to the doctor's treatment of their colleague. This led to a mass signing of an indignant letter from 51 nurses directed at General Hospital School of Nursing, St. John's, Newfoundland. The letter stated that if Miss Southcott and Miss. Redmond resigned as a result of gross insults by Dr. Keegan, the other nurses would also resign.

The second incident occurred a few days later. Florence Scott had graduated from the General Hospital School of Nursing in August of 1913 and left the hospital to work as a private duty nurse in St. John's. In March 1914 she applied for the position of Assistant Superintendent. According to a letter of 30 March 1914 from the Colonial Secretary to Scott, the Governor-in-Council had agreed to the appointment. The records do not show who approached Scott about this position. However, it is clear that Southcott did not recommend or appoint her. As soon as Scott's appointment was made known there was an outcry by the senior nurses on staff and the immediate resignations of three nurses. They maintained they could not work under Scott, a junior nurse whom they had helped train. In addition, they did not think she was competent to fill the position as she had only graduated eight months earlier and, more importantly, they believed that Redmond was entitled to the job after having worked at the General Hospital for so many years.

Keegan added fuel to the fire by informing Southcott that he was going to promote three staff nurses who were resigning. By appointing these three nurses to the positions, Keegan again undermined Southcott's position. Because promotion had always been the right of the Superintendent of Nurses, Southcott refused to recognize these nurses as sisters when they worked on the wards. The feud between Southcott and Keegan was well known by now. Although the nurses wanted the position of sister they would not antagonize Southcott regardless of Keegan, therefore, when they went to work on the wards they did not wear the uniform of a sister. Their loyalty to Southcott and her authority had not been totally diminished. Keegan's action was also in contradiction of the instructions he had received from the Colonial Secretary to maintain all staff in their positions until an Inquiry Board could be formed and the situation reviewed. A Royal commission began its work on 7 May 1914 and took one year to complete. However, many of the members of the board were close allies either to Dr. Keegan or the Conservative Party.

The Commissioners were not medical people and were not familiar with the operation of a hospital and seemed predisposed to support Keegan's point of view. Keegan maintained that the whole problem at the hospital was the fact that there was not one person who was clearly in charge of the institution, and that Southcott was under the delusion that she was in charge of the hospital. He even went so far as to represent Southcott as incompetent, which was soundly refuted by a bevy of witnesses who categorically attested to Southcott's competence and how difficult it was to deal with the obstinate attitude of Dr. Keegan.

A plethora of witnesses, including doctors, supported the view that the Superintendent of Nurses was solely in charge of nurses and nurses' matters. These doctors explained that this was the practice in most hospitals in Canada, the United States and Britain. The doctors almost uniformly stated that Southcott and the nurses ran the hospital efficiently and there had been no friction among the staff until recent months. Most further stated that the Nursing Superintendent should be responsible for nurses promotions and the assignment of their duties.

Southcott submitted evidence to the Commission to show that the general practice in most hospitals was that all nursing staff came under the jurisdiction of the Superintendent of Nurses. Her evidence included letters from nursing superintendents at various hospitals in England, the United States and Canada. Southcott's reputation was reflected in the calibre of the people willing to support her. Yet, it was all for naught, as the outcome was a foregone conclusion, as the all-male Keegan politically allied panel seemed to lend a death ear to those in support of Southcott. The recommendations of the Commission were incorporated into the first General Hospital Act, passed on 15 June 1915 and were subsequently put into place. The General Hospital Act established a rigid staff hierarchy and entrenched the roles of the hospital staff. The Governor-in-Council appointed six businessmen to form the first Board of Governors to administer the hospital and it was made clear that the Superintendent of Nurses would have a much more limited range of duties and the medical superintendent would be the primary authority.

All that Southcott and the nurses had worked for in building the General Hospital School of Nursing disintegrated before their eyes. Southcott continued briefly to fight to retain the little influence she had in the hospital but the Board had other plans. As early as 4 December

1915, the Board of Governors discussed her dismissal. In April 1916 they followed through with this plan and asked for her resignation claiming that "there is no possibility of correcting the trouble so long as Dr. Keegan and Miss Southcott are retained in their present relative positions." Keegan had finally won as control over nursing was taken from the nurses and given to male administrators and doctors. From that point on, the actions by the Board of Governors, on the advice of Dr. Keegan, placed such a strain on the School of Nursing and the nursing staff that by 1924 serious consideration was given to closing the school.[36]

Although most doctors had great respect for Southcott, they still felt that they had to be careful not to go too far in criticizing Keegan, because of his position and political connections. Consequently, Keegan kept firm control and ensured that non-doctors like Southcott did not get too much authority in the hospital. There was no way any politician or doctor could possibly allow a woman, no matter who she was, to assert as much authority as Southcott had.

However, Southcott's battle was an important step in getting recognition for the importance of the nurse and the respect of women in the workplace. She was an inspiration to her fellow nurses and as Linda White points out in *Who's in Charge Here? The General Hospital School of Nursing, St John's, Newfoundland* (White, 1994), that although the episode did not lead to a victory for the nurses, it was just the first in a long-line of steps that made nursing the profession that it is today.

---

[36] Retrieved from
http://www.cbmh.ca/index.php/cbmh/article/viewFile/323/322

Mary Southcott's reputation in the community of St. John's was diminished as a result of this furor. She remained active in nursing and public life for many years. She opened a private maternity hospital and in 1916, the government asked her to take charge of another hospital, established to deal with an epidemic of measles. One of Southcott's assistants in this endeavour was a nurse who had resigned in protest from the General Hospital in 1914.

In addition to her interest in generating more professional respect for nursing, Southcott was an avid suffragette. She organized debates, circulated petitions, and worked diligently with a variety of groups attempting to get the right to vote for women. Throughout this period, Southcott also remained active in the Graduate Nurses' Association and was its president for many years. She died in 1943, but is still fondly remembered to this day as "the Florence Nightingale of Newfoundland."

CHAPTER 7
ISHBEL MARIA HAMILTON-GORDON
IN SERVICE TO SO MANY WHO ARE IN NEED

What does hockey have to do with nursing? Well, let us take a look at a game that was played in 1894 and see how it led to an interest in nursing by a woman who helped found Canada's first order of nurses. The Rideau Hall Rebels, one of Canada's first amateur ice hockey teams, played out of the rink at Rideau Hall, the Ottawa residence of the Governor General Lord Stanley. The team was organized in 1884 by Stanley's third son, Arthur Stanley, and his friend James Creighton, the law clerk of the Senate of Canada, after they had been unceremoniously thrown off the local figure skating rink. The team consisted of young Canadian parliamentarians and government workers, including Stanley's brother William. Creighton, from Darmouth, Nova Scotia, was one of the seven McGill University students who in 1877 invented the seven ice hockey rules that gave the game its first organized structure.

In 1894, Ishbel, Lady Aberdeen, the wife of Stanley's replacement, Lord Aberdeen, witnessed an excetionally rough game on the Rideau Hall rink. She wrote in her journal:

"This game appears to be a most fascinating one and the men get wildly excited about it. But there can be no doubt as to its roughness, and if the players get over keen & lose their tempers as they are too apt to do, the possession of the stick & the close proximity to one another gives the occasion for many a nasty hit. Tonight one man was playing with his nose badly broken & the game had twice to be stopped, once because a man got hit in the mouth &

*the other time because one of the captains was knocked
down unconscious & had to be carried out.* "[37]

What wasn't recorded in her journal was her comment to
a friend that each team needed a nurse to look after the
injured during a game. Her friend replied that there was a
hospital nearby. However, Lady Aberdeen wondered to
herself what recourse players would have if they were
injured in one of the many isolated areas of Canada, where
there were no medical facilities nearby. This concern would
led to an immediate desire to work on ways to bring health
services to the many isolated communities.

Ishbel Maria Hamilton-Gordon was born into a life of
privilege in London, England in 1857. She was the
youngest daughter of Sir Dudley Coutts Marjoribanks, First
Baron of Tweedmouth. Her father was the senior partner in
Coutts Bank and was as noted for his literary and artistic
tastes as for his business acumen.

One evening in the summer of 1868, a young sportsman
lost his way in the wild district around the Marjoribanks'
country estate and begged for shelter at the home of Sir
Dudley. Marjoribanks welcomed the youthful sportsman,
who was the Earl of Aberdeen. When the 11 year old Ishbel
saw the young nobleman, she was immediately taken by his
handsome bearing. Though too young at the time for a
romantic attachment, this first meeting led to admiration
between Lord Aberdeen and Miss Marjoribanks that
flowered into a romantic attachment as she grew older, and
in 1877, as Lady Aberdeen, she was married to Lord
Aberdeen and left her father's home to go and preside at

---

[37] Reprieved from http://canadachannel.ca/HCO/index.php/1894_-
Lady_Abberdeen_ watches_a_Hockey_Game_at_Rideau_Hall

Haddo House in Aberdeen, Scotland. Both of them resolved to devote their lives to meaningful work which should do something positive for those who seemed put upon by a system that only rewarded those at the top.

Her penchant for the nursing arts was formulated at a young age when she was a volunteer in the slums of Aberdeen, working with tuberculosis victims, much to the chagrin of her upper-class friends who thought it appalling that she would subject herself to such demeaning work. It was at the same time that she helped found the National Council of Women to assist prostitutes in breaking free of the streets. Her work was not interrupted by her marriage or children, but it did put a strain on her as she had to juggle her duties as the wife of an aristocrat and the mother of five children while continuing her commitment to social justice and health care for those least likely to receive either.

Ishbel started the Haddo House Association, which was founded on democratic principles and promoted a system of equality for all. Her own servants were urged to join and to take part in classes for singing, drawing and wood-carving. She encouraged them to band together in order to assure they were all being properly treated by her, her husband and those in charge of their daily routines. She arranged lectures and cultural events especially for them. This social effort gradually spread far beyond the Aberdeen estate, and eventually became *The Onward and Upward Association*, which had branches throughout Scotland and eventually the rest of England.

This tireless effort in pursuit of social justice and the physical well-being of the less fortunate was in one way, no doubt, an effort to assuage the deep depression she was suffering from the loss of her youngest child. Although supportive of her work, Lord Aberdeen began to sense that she needed to relinquish some of her commitments. Yet, she steadfastly refused. Eventually, she had a nervous breakdown in the late 1880's. Struggling to overcome the debilitating illness, Ishbel became friends with the nurse who looked after her. This friendship made her realize the importance of nurses to the physical well-being of a patient, but she also became more cognizant of how important they were to the emotional stability that was also critical to a patient's recovery. Her respect and admiration grew for nurses who reached out with the hand of compassion to those suffering physical and mental anguish.

In spite of her illness, she was appalled by the poverty of the country, and she used all her energies and influence to get a market for the beautiful woven materials, the exquisite laces and the dainty carvings manufactured in cottages and convents all across the countryside, primarily by Irish immigrants. She formed the *Irish Industries Association* to market the goods produced by those who struggled for survival in a economic system much like today's, where all the benefits seemed to flow to those at the top. Shops were opened in London and Dublin and other large provincial towns, and the goods brought to the notice of the public, and all the profits went directly to the workers without middlemen or some corporate entity skimming most of the money off the top.

Yet, all this activity could not diminish her deep depression. For that reason, Lord Aberdeen sought a position that would allow them to leave the U.K. in hopes that new surroundings might lift her spirits. Thus, he eagerly accepted an appointment as Governor General of Canada in 1893. The five years in Canada were fruitful years for Ishbel. Upon arrival, Ishbel thought it would be better not to connect herself directly with any women's organization, and so she resolved to watch and learn something of the ways of the new country before attempting any practical effort. The result of this experiment Ishbel tells in her own words: "Within a month of our landing, a meeting was convened to form a National Council of Women of Canada to bind together in mutual aid and sympathy the workers in connection with every society of national interest in the Dominion, without distinction of religious or political views. Despite my newly formed resolution, I felt impelled to join in organizing the Council, and now I can never be sufficiently thankful for the intercourse which it gave me with noble women of every class, and every creed, who were all labouring for the common weal."[38]

In her duties at Ottawa's Government House, invitations were eagerly sought to state dinners where she became famous for dramatizing incidents in Canadian history, using household staff, guests and family members to play roles. She and Lord Aberdeen, spent their own money to stage a huge pageant in Toronto celebrating Canada's progress in industry, arts, sciences and sports. Their willingness to recognize Canadian uniqueness endeared them to the citizens.

Nurses, doctors and hospitals were desperately needed in remote areas of Canada at the time, as well as in rapidly growing towns and cities. In 1897 to commemorate Queen Victoria's Diamond Jubilee, Lady Aberdeen organized the Victorian Order of Nurses. How this came about is a

---

[38] Retrieved from http://www.electricsscotland.com/history/decendents/chap32.htm

testament to Ishbel's steadfast dedication and determination to see that healthcare was available to all citizens as a human right, long before Tommy Douglas enshrined the idea of universal, free healthcare as a part of the Canadian psyche.

The idea for the order germinated when Lady Aberdeen was a participant at the annual meeting in Halifax of the *National Council of Women*, where horror stories were exchanged by the women in attendance about the abysmal state of healthcare in many parts of Canada. In her autobiography, VON's founder was later to write of this meeting:

" ...many of the members told pathetic stories of cases where young mothers and children had died, whilst husbands and fathers were traveling many weary miles for the medical and nursing aid which might have saved them..." [39]

Lady Aberdeen was asked by the group to found an order of visiting nurses in Canada. The order was to be a memorial to the 60th anniversary of Queen Victoria's ascent to the throne of the British Empire. At a Rideau Hall meeting on February 10, 1897, Prime Minister Sir Wilfrid Laurier offered the motion inaugurating the Victorian Order of Nurses for Canada. When criticism from Canada's medical establishment caused Parliamentary support to falter, Ishbel appealed to the children of Canada for help, writing to their schools about the need for nurses to care for sick people in their own homes. She encouraged them to flood Parliament with letters of support for the VON. Below is part of the letter she sent that was read to

---

[39] Retrieved from http://www.von.ca/en/about/history.aspx

virtually every school child in Canada, appealing to them to support the VON.

"In the towns they will go to those who cannot now afford the care of trained nurses and often die for lack of it.."

"On the prairies, in the forests, in mining districts - - everywhere throughout the country - - they will go hither and thither amongst our brave pioneers and bring help to these heroic people who are building up the future of this beautiful country amidst many hardships and privations..." [40]

Ishbel, appointed first president of VON, enlisted the help of Dr. Alfred Worcester, professor of hygiene at Harvard University and founder of the Waltham Training School for District Nurses in Massachusetts, to help promote VON. Dr. Worcester explained the importance and potential of the district nursing idea to large numbers throughout Canada. He also encouraged Miss Charlotte Macleod, superintendent of the Waltham school, to come to Ottawa and help set up VON. Miss Macleod, a Canadian who had studied with the legendary Florence Nightingale, became VON's first chief superintendent.

VON's first 12 nurses were admitted to the order at a ceremony in November 1897, and soon thereafter, Queen Victoria granted the organization its royal charter.

To understand the importance of Ishbel's founding of the order, it is necessary to explore the order's significance in the development of nursing as a respected and revered profession in Canada. For that, we were delighted to glean

---

[40] Retrieved from http://www.von.ca/en/about/history.aspx

some of the highlights from VON's history in regards to its significant contributions to Canadian healthcare.

The initial aims of the order were to provide visiting nursing services to districts without access to medical facilities and to establish cottage hospitals in isolated areas. The VON established 44 such hospitals in local communities and within isolated areas throughout Canada. Responsibility for running these institutions was gradually assumed by community groups, with the last VON-run hospital being placed in the hands of local citizens in 1924. Since then the functions of the VON have evolved in response to changes in Canadian society and new home-nursing needs. More recent initiatives include home-based palliative care, adult day programs, foot-care clinics, respite care, primary health care clinics and health services in shelters for women, children and youth at risk.

The story of the Victorian Order of Nurses is a vital part of the very history of Canada itself and its early expansion and social development, and of its changing ideals through two world wars, a great depression and the introduction of new medical technologies.[41]

For nearly 125 years, VON has pioneered health services in Canada. It has a proud tradition of often being the first to identify emerging health and social needs, and then providing innovative services that meet those needs.

In 1898, Charlotte Macleod directed the formation of a team of four nurses to accompany the Canadian Field Force, an expedition of military and government officials, to the Klondike region of what is now the Yukon Territory.

---

[41] Retrieved from http://www.von.ca/en/about/history.aspx

Although this was the year Lady Aberdeen left Canada, it was she who was the driving force behind VON, so it was through her efforts in founding the order that the story of the Klondike nurses can be told. These nurses' exploits in providing care to the miners during the gold rush, under the most difficult of conditions, became one of the earliest epic tales in VON's long and colourful history.

Lady Aberdeen helped organize VON recruitment sites in the cities of Ottawa, Montreal, Toronto, Halifax, Vancouver and Kingston. Through the Boar War, two world wars, the Korean conflict and many Canadian disasters, the VON has been devoted to meeting the changing health care needs of Canadian society. VON Canada continues to be a dynamic and responsive organization. Canadians owe a debt of gratitude to Ishbel Maria Hamilton-Gordon for having the foresight to found this compassionate organization dedicated to serving the healthcare needs of Canadians.[42]

Ishbel Maria Hamilton-Gordon continued her commitment to social causes after returning to Scotland, but she shall always be fondly remembered in Canada for founding the Victorian Order of Nurses that continues to this day in service to so many who are in need.

---

[42] Retrieved from
http://www.electricscotland.com/history/descendants/chap32.htm

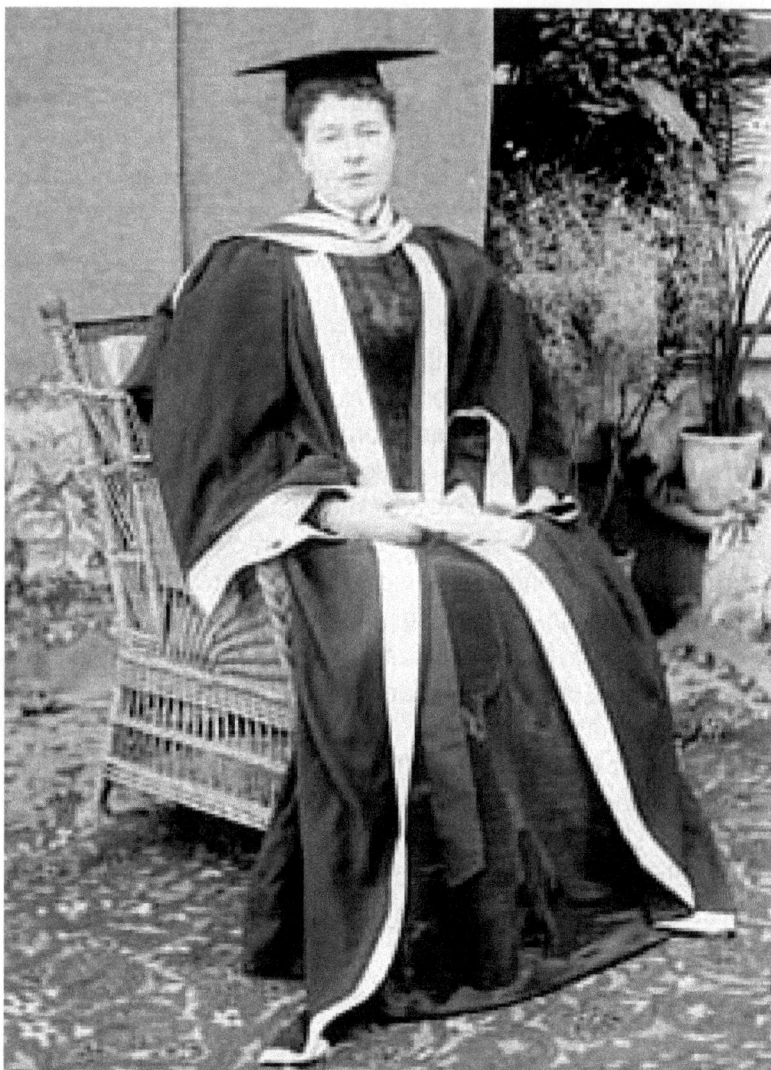

Lady Aberdeen was the first woman to receive an honorary degree in Canada. She is shown here in Queen's University robes, photographed by William James Topley. [43]

---

[43] Retrieved from http://en.wikipedia.org/wiki/Ishbel_Hamilton-Gordon,_Marchioness _of_Aberdeen_and_Temair

SERVICES PROVIDED
BY
THE VICTORIAN ORDER OF NURSES TODAY [44]

Personal Services

Care-giving Support
Children's Services
Community Support Services
Crisis Services
Custom Care
Foot Care Services
Health Promotion and Education Services
Immunization Services
Mental health Services
Nursing and Professional Services
Occupational Services
Palliative Care Services
Personal Support/Home Support
Special Services

Corporate Health and Wellness

Institutional Health
Seasonal Flu
Workplace Wellness

Special Projects

Aboriginal Health Initiatives
Assembly of First Nations
Fetal Alcohol Syndrome (FASD)
Healthy Baby and Me

---

[44] Retrieved from http://www.von.ca/en/careers/careers.aspx

Healthy Workplace for Home and Community Care Nurses
Pharmaceutical Support Services
Reach Up and Reach-Out
SMART Program
SMILE Program

CHAPTER 8
MYRA BENNETT AND THE GREEN HOUSE OF MERCY

There is a green house in Daniel's Harbour, Newfoundland that is a national heritage sight. It is a monument to Myra Bennett who devoted her life to caring for people along the coast of Newfoundland. Bennett was simply know throughout the 300 kilometres of the coast that she served as "the nurse." Like Mary Meagre Southcott, she was sometimes referred to as "the Florence Nightingale of Newfoundland." Regardless of what she was called, she was the only medical professional for most people who lived along the isolated stretch of Newfoundland's coast. Though she is slightly out of the time-frame for this book, it is important to mention her as an example of nurses who were determined angels of mercy serving valiantly in difficult circumstances in often primitive conditions in isolated places.

Born in London, England, in 1890, Myra Bennett served as a nurse in England for 10 years before coming to Newfoundland in 1921. She was persuaded to move to Newfoundland by Lady Harris, the wife of Sir Alexander Harris, Governor of Newfoundland at that time. Told of the dire need of her services, Myra accepted a two-year contract that paid her $75 per month ($900 per year). During her first year there, she met and married local ex-merchant marine Angus Bennett, and in 1922 they moved into the house he had built. The home soon became the place everyone went when they were having medical difficulties.

Bennett's medical career along that stretch of coast became the stuff of legends. Daniel's Harbour was an isolated community at that time. There were no roads or railway connecting the community to the outside world. There was a coastal steamer, but it operated only in good weather. The nearest hospital was the Grenfell Mission, established in St. Anthony, several hundred kilometres to the north.

During Bennett's tenure she estimated that she delivered 5,000 babies and extracted 3,000 teeth. Her greatest feat of medical skill came in 1926 when her brother-in-law, Alex, slipped and fell into the teeth of a lumber saw and almost severed his foot. Cleaning up the wound as best she could, Bennett proceeded to stitch the severed foot back onto the leg. She did such a good job that he kept his foot at a time when the reattachment of limbs was rarely, if ever, considered medically feasible. When doctors learned what she did, her procedure was written up in a medical journal.

She officially retired in 1953, but she continued to assist people whenever she was asked. During Bennett's life she received an honorary doctorate from Memorial University; she was the subject of a *Reader's Digest* article, a CBC-TV documentary called "Lady of the Lonely Places" and a book by H. Gordon Green called *Don't Have Your Baby in the Dory*.[45] Bennett passed away in 1990 at the age of 100. In 1993 the house was no longer occupied after the death of her husband, Angus, at the age of 96. It is now a heritage sight. Though her memory may be fading with time, her residence is still known as the little green house of mercy.

---

[45] Retrieved from
http://www.heritage.nf.ca/society/rhs/cf_listing/043.html

Awards Received by Myra Bennett[46]

1935 - King George V Silver Jubilee Medal

1936 - Member of the Order of the British Empire

1937 - King George VI Coronation Medal

1957 - Queen Elizabeth II Coronation Medal

1967 - Honorary Membership Associarion for Registered Nurses

1974 - Member of the Order of Canada

1974 - Doctor of Science, Memorial University

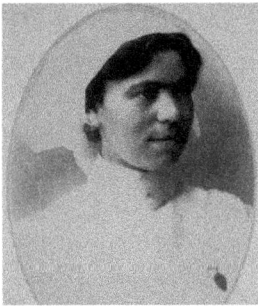

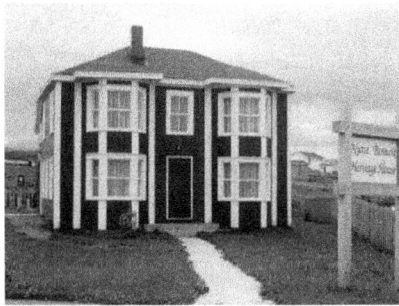

Myra Bennett[47] (Circa 1923)
and The Green House of Mercy Memorial[48]

---

[46] Retrieved from http://en.wikipedia.org/wiki/Myra_Bennett
[47] Retrieved from http://www.facebook.com/photo.php?fbid =161161463921477&set
[48] Retrieved from http://www.heritage.nf.ca/society/rhs/cf_listing/043.html

CHAPTER 9
IT WAS OUR DUTY AS CANADIANS

Nurses had served in the Canadian Army Medical Corps since the 1885 Northwest Rebellion and compiled a distinguished record during the South African Boar War (1899-1902). The Canadian Army Nursing Corps was established in 1908, but had only five permanent members by the start of the World War I. In August 1914, the Matron-in-Chief, Major Margaret Macdonald, an experienced nurse who had served in South Africa, received permission to enlist 100 nurses. Almost all were drawn from hospitals, universities, and medical professions from across Canada.

In September of 1914, 105 Canadian nurses sailed to England as part of the first contingent of soldiers sent to aid the war effort. By 1918, the number of nurses serving had grown to over 3,000. All of them were volunteers. Called "Bluebirds" by the soldiers, because of their blue dresses, they served in medical facilities and combat aid stations in France, Belgium, Greece, Malta and the Eastern Mediterranean.[49]

World War I was often referred to as a meat-grinder, because never before had technology been used on such a large scale for the literal slaughter of not only soldiers, but vast civilian populations that got caught in the cross-fire. Canadian nurses offered compassionate care to all who fell before this tirade of terror. Called nursing sisters, because some of the earliest nurses belonged to religious orders, they were accorded the rank of lieutenant. Most worked in military hospitals or at special aid stations near the front

---

[49] Retrieved from
http://www.warmuseum.ca/cwm/exhibitions/guerre/nurses-e.aspx

lines. World War I marked the first time that they would incur casualties. Although hospitals were supposed to be accorded safe status by both sides, there were many bombing incidents, particularly as stalemate set-in and both sides often resorted to barbaric acts. One of these acts was committed toward the end of the war, on 19 May 1918, when the Germans bombed the Canadian General Hospital at Étaples, France.

Étaples was the scene of much Allied activity during World War I due to its safety from attack by enemy land forces and the existence of railway connections with both the northern and southern battlefields. The town was home to 16 hospitals and a convalescent depot, in addition to a number of reinforcement camps for Commonwealth soldiers and general barracks for the French Army. Over 10,000 men died in battles around Étaples.

The abundance of military infrastructure in Étaples gave the town a capacity of around 100,000 troops and made the area a serious target for German aerial bombing raids, from which the town suffered heavily. It appears that Commonwealth authorities made no attempt to segregate the troop staging areas from the hospitals or civilian areas. For that reason, it was often difficult for Germans to avoid colateral damage to hospitals and civilian areas when conducting bombing. When the Canadian hospital was bombed, one nurse was killed and seven others injured. The war would rage on for six more months, and this would not be the last time a hospital was bombed.

The dangers for nurses was not limited to the land. One of the innovations of the First World War Medical Services was the introduction of the hospital ship, used to evacuate the sick and wounded back to Canada. These ships were also subject to enemy attack such as occurred on the night of 27 June 1917. The *Llandovery Castle*, a British merchant vessel serving as a Canadian hospital ship, was torpedoed while returning to Liverpool, England from Halifax, Nova Scotia. Of a Canadian crew and medical staff totalling 258, only twenty-four survived. Among those who perished were the fourteen Canadian nurses aboard. Several nurses had escaped on lifeboats but were machine-gunned by a German U-boat.

As patients arrived by truck or rail, the nurses were among the first to meet wounded soldiers, cleaning wounds and offering comfort. They assisted in surgery and often had primary responsibility for cleaning post-surgical wounds and watching for secondary infections. Nurses cared for wounds daily, bandaging and re-bandaging injuries and ensuring that oxygen entered wounds to destroy the anaerobic infections that could result in a patient's painful death.[50]

Of the approximately 3000 Canadian nurses who served overseas, 49 were killed from enemy fire, disease, or drowning during the war. Nurses returned from overseas with refined medical skills that infused their profession with new medical techniques and a heightened sense of legitimacy. They had won the affection of thousands of Canadian soldiers who often referred to them as "Sisters of Mercy" or "Angels of Mercy." A memorial to the war's nurses was erected in Ottawa in 1926 in the Parliament of Canada's Hall of Honour.[51] (See page 105)

---

[50] Retrieved from
http://www.warmuseum.ca/cwm/exhibitions/guerre/nurses-e.aspx
[51] Retrieved from http://www.heroines.ca/celebrate/statuenursing.html

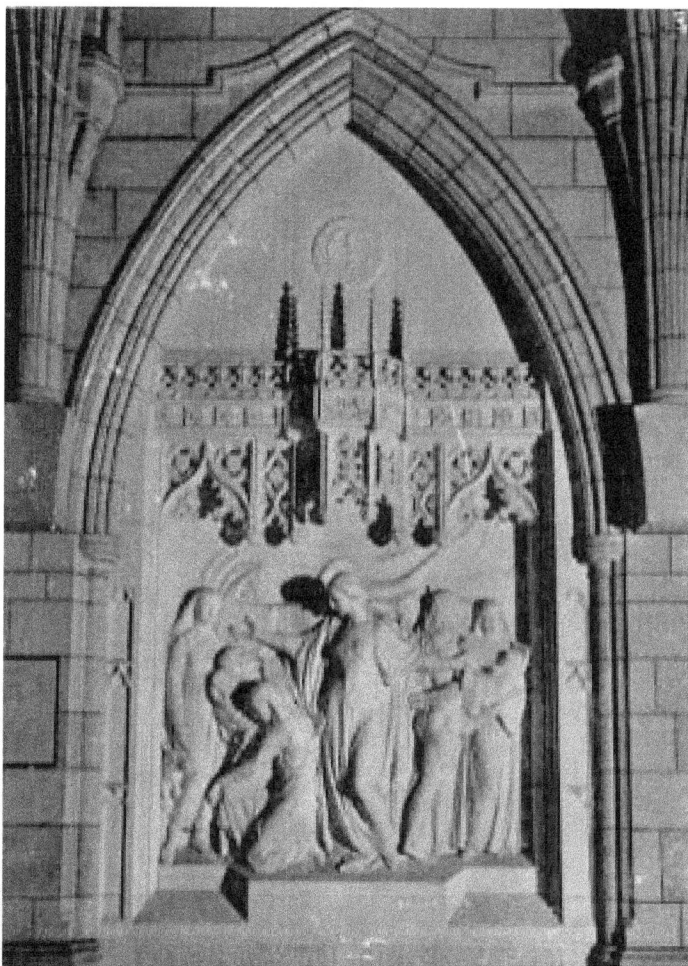

The above Canadian Nursing Sister's Memorial commemorates the contribution of nurses in Canada from the earliest days until World War I. The panel is mounted in the Parliament Buildings in Ottawa, Ontario in the Hall of Honour located in the Centre Block. Montreal artist G.W. Hill sculpted the panel from marble in Carara, Italy. The figures on the right-hand side are a nurse in New France caring for a native child while an Iroquois warrior looks on. The central figure is intended to represent humanity, while the group at left features two uniformed nurses from World War I.

Designed by Vernon March in the mid 1920s, Canada's National War Memorial dedicated to those who served in World War I, also known as *The Response*, is among the first to commemorate both male and female service persons in a single monument. The nurse is clearly visible in the section from the monument pictured below.[52]

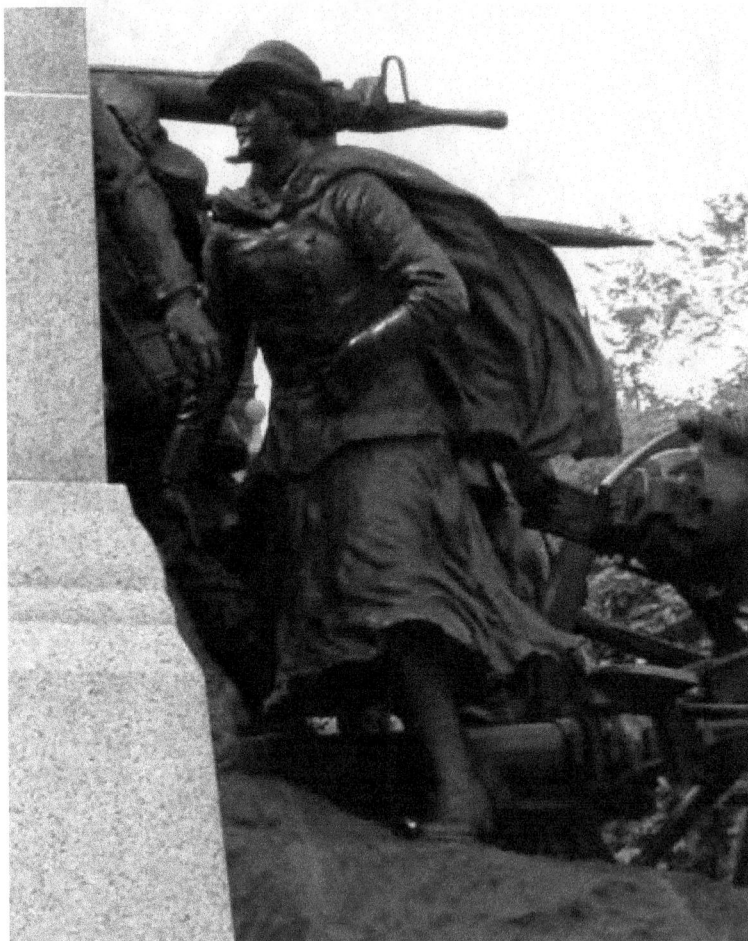

---

[52] Retrieved from http://www.museevirtuel-virtualmuseum.ca/sgc-cms/expositions-exhibitions/tresors-treasures/?page_id=7469&lang=en

The memorials are a fitting tribute to the Canadian nurses of World War I, who served valiantly alongside men. For too long, war memorials had only glamorized wars and the men who fought them, but both of these memorials showed the personal agony endured by those who had to face death on the far-flung battlefields of a merciless conflict. Further, they included women for the first time, as willing but beleaguered participants, who shouldered the duty of caring for those who were felled in battle. For the first time, women were an important part of the historical narrative of war.

The personal histories of the 47 dedicated, brave nurses who made the ultimate sacrifice in World War I are varied, but they all had a common goal to reach out with compassion to those who needed assistance, and many times, this included enemy soldiers as well as their Canadian brethren. Their greatest loss at one time occurred when the Llandovery Castle hospital ship was sunk by a German U-boat. All 14 nurses aboard perished on 27 June 1918.

I. The Sinking of the Llandovery Castle

The information that follows is a descriptive account of the personal interviews officials had with the survivors of the sinking of the hospital ship Llandovery Castle and affords convincing evidence of the deliberate intent of the German U-boat captain to ignore the rules of war and the Geneva Convention in regards to non-combatants and hospital ships. Furthermore, it is an example of true professionalism and courage under fire by 14 women who were unwilling to yield to fear. To this very day, the sinking of the Llandovery Castle remains one of the most heinous atrocities committed in war.

How the Nurses Died

"Unflinchingly and calmly, as steady and collected as if on parade, without a complaint or a single sign of emotion, our fourteen devoted nursing sisters faced the terrible ordeal of certain death, only a matter of minutes, as our lifeboat neared that mad whirlpool of waters where all human power was helpless."[53]

The above is an excerpt from Sergeant A. Knight's story of the destruction of the Llandovery Castle. Official verification of the facts surrounding the sinking of H.M.H.S. Llandovery Castle indicate it was a dastardly act perpetrated by the German captain and his underlings who completely disregarded the rules of engagement and respect for the Red Cross insignia that was displayed on the ship.

Deliberate Murders:

It is not known whether the German captain realized his crime before or after torpedoing the ship. However, what is obvious was the attempt to cover it up by ramming, shelling and sinking the life-boats with 258 survivors of the sinking. Somehow, one boat containing twenty-four survivors, managed to escape the carnage. Obviously, if there were no survivors, there would be no one who could testify about the German U-Boat captain's disregard for the rules of engagement.

The survivors recounted a stirring story of the perfect discipline and bravery exhibited by the fourteen nurses who valiantly tried to administer first aid while the ship was

---

[53] Retrieved from
http://www.waramps.ca/uploadedFiles/English_Site/Military_Heritage

sinking, many refusing to board the lifeboats so they could tend the injured on the decks of the ship. Many of the nurses were veterans who had served on the western front in France as early as 1914.

How magnificently they faced the final ordeal on that awful evening of 27 June 1918, is simply, yet graphically, related in the story of Sergeant A. Knight, the non-commissioned officer of the Llandovery Castle, who took charge of life-boat No. 5, into which the fourteen nurses were finally placed after the injured had been put on another boat.[54]

"Our boat," said Sergeant Knight, "was quickly loaded and lowered to the surface of the water. Then the crew of eight men and myself faced the difficulty of getting free from the ropes holding us to the ship's side. I broke two axes trying to cut ourselves away, but was unsuccessful. With the forward motion and choppy sea the boat all the time was pounding against the ship's side. To save the boat we tried to keep ourselves away by using the oars, and soon every one of the latter were broken. Finally the ropes became loose at the top and we commenced to drift away. We were carried towards the stern of the ship, when suddenly the poop-deck seemed to break away and sink. The suction drew us quickly into the vacuum, the boat tipped over sideways, and every occupant went under. I estimate we were together in the boat about eight minutes. In that whole time I did not hear a complaint or murmur from one of the nurses. There was not a cry for help or any outward evidence of fear. In the entire time I overheard

---

[54] Retrieved from
http://www.waramps.ca/uploadedFiles/English_Site/Military_Heritage/Media/PDF/inff.pdf

only one remark when the matron, Nursing Sister M.M. Fraser, turned to me as we drifted helplessly towards the stern of the ship and asked if there was any hope for survival. I replied negatively, seeing myself our helplessness without oars and the sinking condition of the stern of the ship. A few seconds later we were drawn into the whirlpool of the submerged afterdeck, and the last I saw of the nursing sisters was as they were thrown over the side of the boat. All were wearing life-belts."

"It was," concluded Sergeant Knight, "doubtful if any of them came to the surface again, although I myself sank and came up three times, finally clinging to a piece of wreckage and being eventually picked up by the captain's boat."[55]

II. Honour Roll of Nurses Who Perished in the Llandovery Castle

Let us review the brief histories of the nurses who perished in the sinking of the Llandovery Castle.

Mae Sampson

A story in the 6 July 1918 edition of the *Collingwood Messenger* bore the headline "Nurse Sampson Lost on Hospital Ship," and indicated her mother and cousin, who lived in Toronto, received a letter from Sampson from Halifax stating she was sailing the next trip to Liverpool.

Sampson was 28 when she died. She trained at the Hamilton, Ontario Hospital and became a private nurse for 3 years before becoming the first nurse from Hamilton to enlist in 1914. She spent most of her time on the western

---

[55] Retrieved from http://www.gwpda.org/naval/lcastl11.htm

front in France and in the muddy, disease laden fields of Flanders in Belgium. She attended to King George V after he was injured on the front lines, even going so far as to accompany him back to England when he insisted he wanted her by his side on the trip. She was decorated for bravery before being transferred to the hospital in Salonika, Greece.

A series of circumstances would lead to her winding up on the Llandovery castle. Sampson fell ill with diphtheria in October 1917 and was sent back to England for recuperation. She then returned to Canada for a short leave. She was anxious to return to duty and volunteered for hospital ship duty on the first vessel available, which happened to be the Llandovery Castle.

Today, the Hamilton Hospital's roll of honour has the following inscription on it in regards to Sampson: "To the glory of God and in honoured memory of Nursing Sister Mae Belle Sampson, C.A.M.C., who made the supreme sacrifice in the sinking of the S.S. Llandovery Castle, June 27, 1918. Her soul liveth!" [56]

Margaret Marjory Fraser

Margaret was born in New Glasgow, Nova Scotia in 1885, and was the daughter of Duncan Cameron Fraser who was Lieutenant Governor of Nova Scotia, a member of the Canadian Parliament and a Nova Scotia Supreme Court Justice. Only a few months before her death, her brother was killed on the western front of France. She was 33 years old when she died.

---

[56] Retrieved from
http://www.theenterprisebulletin.com/ArticleDisplay.aspex=3357746

Christina Campbell

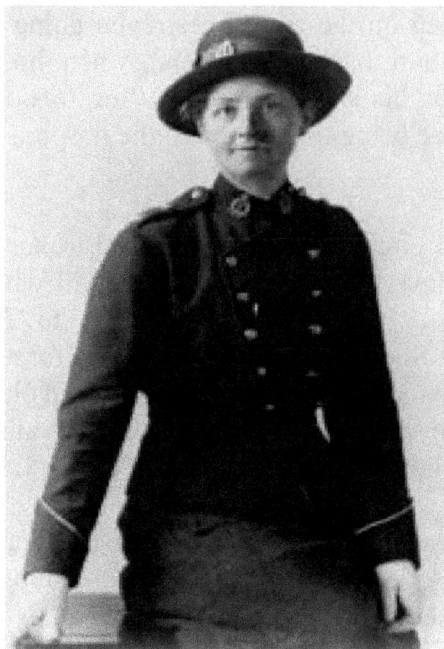

Christina Campbell – 1916 [57]

Christina Campbell was born in Inverness, Scotland on 17 August 1877. Leaving her parents and three sisters behind, at the age of 16, she joined her brother Angus in Victoria, British Columbia. Four years later, she graduated from the Royal Jubilee Hospital of Nursing and continued to work with great distinction in Victoria until 1915, when she joined the Canadian Army Medical Corps. She took a cut in pay in order to serve, as her salary in the CMAC was $50 per month. She was assigned to the #2 Canadian General Hospital, a tent hospital of over 1,000 beds, in

---

[57] Retrieved from http://camc.wordpress.com/2010/01/22/nursing-sister-christina-campbell/

France. As many as 500 soldiers a day arrived in convoys and all had to be received, diagnosed, and allocated to wards with minimal delay.

The work was relentless and the conditions challenging. By mid November Christina was transferred back to London and then to the medical evacuation force, where she worked ferrying the wounded to hospitals in England until June 1916, when she was transferred to Malta. This assignment was cut short when she became ill and was sent to England for recuperation.

In August 1917 Christina was reassigned to the Eye and Ear Hospital in Westcliffe in the UK, where she stayed until March 1918 when she was posted to transport duty on the Canadian hospital ship the Llandovery Castle. Hospital ship assignment was considered an easy posting and was often given as a reward to overworked nurses. The assignment entailed caring for the injured soldiers who were being shipped home to Halifax for convalescence, further medical attention or medical discharge. On the return journey, the Canadian doctors and nurses could enjoy the relaxing sea voyage under the hospital ship lights and designation, which by international agreement, protected them from enemy attack. After 2 1/2 years of active war service, Christina probably looked forward to the slower pace of hospital ship life. The peacefulness was shattered on 27 June 1918.

Christina Campbell's name is commemorated in the First World War Book of Remembrance held in Ottawa and her name is also inscribed on the Halifax Memorial in Nova Scotia's capital. Standing in Point Pleasant Park, the 12 metre high Cross of Sacrifice is visible to all ships approaching the Halifax Harbour. It stands as a memorial to the over 3000 Canadian men and women who lost their lives at sea in the service of their country during the two world wars. The inscription reads: "Their graves are unknown but their memory shall endure."[58]

Carola Josephine Douglas

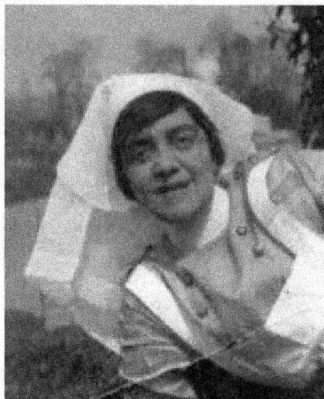

Born in 1887 in Toronto, Carola enlisted in the Canadian Army Medical Corps in early 1915. She was assigned to Étaples, where she worked at No. 2 Canadian General Hospital. In October 1915 she was assigned to the No. 2 British Stationary Hospital at Abbeville for short term temporary assignment. She was returned to Étaples and given three days leave.

In November of 1916, she was transferred to Salonika, where several of the others nurses who eventually wound up on the Llandovery Castle also served at various times. In March 1917, she suffered from badly infected fingers, a potentially life-threatening injury at the time. She recovered and returned to duty. However, by October 1917, she was

---

[58] Retrieved from www.bcnursinghistory.ca/cmss/uploads/Christina Campbell%20%20Tragedy%20%20%of20%20%the20%Llandovery %20%20Castle.pdf

exhausted from overwork and stress. She was sent back to England, where she was admitted to the Canadian Red Cross Special Hospital in Basingstoke to rest and recuperate. After her health was restored, Carola was attached to No. 16 Canadian General Hospital in Orpington, Kent. In March 1918, she too was transferred to the Llandovery Castle, where she would share the same fate as the other nurses on that ship.[59] Upon boarding the ship, she looked out at the ocean that lay before her and was rumoured to have said "I can't believe how much I miss being with our brave lads"

Anna Irene Stamers

The military file on Anna Irene Stamers is a thick one. It describes a slender brown haired woman with blue eyes, standing 5' 6 1/2 inches tall. Anna was from St. John, New Brunswick. At the time of enlistment on 3 June 1915, she was living at 171 Waterloo Street with her widowed mother, Sarah Stamers. Her service record describes Anna as having been assigned to No. 1 General Hospital in Étaples. Like so many nurses, Anna faced the risk of catching illnesses from the patients she served. Just four months after arrival, she became a patient, as she contracted a serious infection. In July she returned to duty in England where she was ultimately transferred to the Ontario Military Hospital in Orpington, Kent. In March 1918, she was transferred to the Llandovery Castle. After an uneventful journey to Canada, caring for wounded men returning home, she enjoyed a short leave. In July, she boarded the ship for the return journey. Sadly, she didn't

---

[59] Retrieved from
http://rememberingfirstworldwarnurses.blogspot.com/2010/10/-carola-douglas-and-anna.html

make it back to England. Her records are simply stamped "Missing, Believed Drowned."[60]

Alexina Dussault

Alexina was a Montreal native and a graduate of the Royal Victoria Hospital nursing program. She enlisted in September 1914, and had served on several hospital ships, including the Araguaya and the Letitia (both in 1917). Alexina had also served in France at No. 2 Canadian Stationary Hospital and at the Ontario Military Hospital in Orpington, Kent.

Alexina was always eager to volunteer for duty on hospital ships. She was excited about the voyage on the Llandovery Castle, as she knew several of the soldiers on board. It is rumoured that her last words before sailing were, "I can't believe how lucky I am to be sailing on this ship."

Minnie Asenath Follette

Born 11 November 1884 in Port Greville, Nova Scotia, she enlisted in 1911 and in 1914 volunteered for duty at the 1st Canadian Casualty Station in France. Working continuously for nearly two years without leave, she was sent to England for two months rest, where she immediately got out of bed and assisted her fellow nurses who were caring for the severely disabled soldiers who were being sent there for convalescent care. In August of 1917, she was posted to the HMS Letita hospital ship for three months. Then, to the Ontario Military Hospital in

---

[60] Retrieved from
http://rememberingfirstworldwarnurses.blogspot.com/2010/10-anna

Kent, England where her superiors thought she would get more rest. She pleaded for a return to the front, but in March of 1918 she was posted to the Llandovery Castle. Her military decorations included the two Gold Stars, British War Medal, Victory Medal, Memorial Plaque, Memorial Scroll and the Memorial Cross. One soldier said of her, "day or night, when you opened your eyes, there she was with her wonderful smile, making you realize that someone genuinely cared about you."

Margaret Jane Fortescue

Born in York Factory, Manitoba in 1878, near what is now Churchill, Margaret Jane was descended from a historic Canadian family. Her father was Joseph Fortescue, Chief Factor for the Hudson Bay Company at York Factory from 1872-1884. Her father died in 1899. Having depended on him for support since she served as his aid, she opted for the new profession of nursing, graduating from the Montreal General Hospital School of Nursing in 1905.

On April 22, 1915, Margaret enlisted with the Canadian Army Medical Corps. She was assigned to Number 3 Canadian General Hospital in Camiers, France. Her unit arrived in England on May 15 and was sent to France on 16 June. She also served in Boulogne, when the unit was transferred there.

In 1916, one of her brothers died of tuberculosis. Perhaps that news, together with the intense strain of the work at the overwhelmed hospital in Boulogne contributed to Margaret's first of many work-related illnesses. In January of 1917, she was suffering from bronchitis and given three weeks sick leave to England. Following this illness, she returned to Carmiers. In February 1918, she was sick again with bronchitis. She was treated at Wimereaux, France and then recovered at a British convalescent home in London. Finally, on 10 April 1918, she was discharged and given a lighter assignment. She was assigned to the Llandovery Castle.

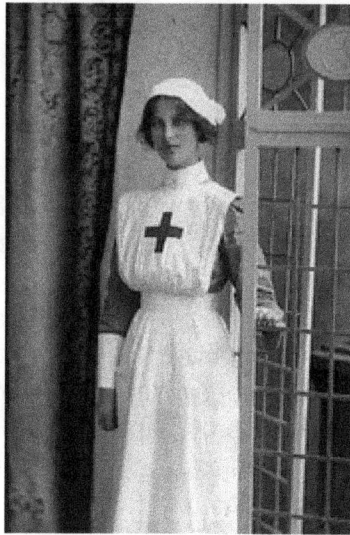

Margaret Jane Fortescue
at Carmiers, France 1916[61]

Minnie Katherine Gallaher

Born in Pittsburg, Ontario on 1 January 1880, she enlisted in 1915 and was dispatched to a front line hospital in France where she served with great distinction for three years. Exhausted from overwork, she was transferred to

[61] Retrieved from http://www.rememberingfirstworldwarnurses.blogs pot.com/2011/02

what was considered lighter duty and assigned to the Llandovery Castle hospital ship. When the Llandovery Castle left Halifax for Liverpool, the final words she wrote her mother were, "I am in a safe avenue now, so do not worry."

Jessie Mabel McDiarmid

Jessie was born on a ranch in Ashton, Ontario, but her enlistment records indicate no date of birth. She enlisted in 1915 in London, Ontario and spent nearly three years at front line hospitals. Her reputation for efficiency and compassion were well documented by many soldiers in her care. Like several other nurses, she was assigned to hospital ships to lighten her duties. That is why she was on the Llandovery Castle.

Mary Agnes McKenzie

Mary Agnes McKenzie was born 28 April 1880 in Toronto, Ontario to
Scottish immigrant parents. She took her nursing studies at the Rochester General Hospital and graduated in 1903. She enlisted in January of 1916. Mary's first posting overseas was to the Ontario Military Hospital at Kent, England. However, she must have wanted to return home for a visit in 1918. That led to her assignment to the Llandovery Castle for its return to Liverpool, England.

Rena McLean

Born in New Brunswick in 1879, Rena attended college and then studied nursing at a Rhode Island Hospital, graduating in 1908. She was a head nurse at a Massachusetts hospital until September of 1914 when she enlisted in the Canadian Medical Corps. Once in France, she helped with the conversion of a hotel into a Canadian hospital and served in a variety of field hospitals until March of 1918 when she was assigned to the Llandovery Castle.

Gladys Irene Sare

Born in 1889, Gladys enlisted in 1916 in Montreal and served in France and on several hospital ships in addition to the Llandovery castle. Known for a vivacious smile and usually the tallest female (5:10) in the CMC, she was described by one soldier as "a ray of sunshine in a place of gloom."

Jean Templeman

Born in Ottawa in 1885, Jean enlisted in Montreal in 1915. While Gladys Sare was 5:10, Jean was a diminutive 4:11, and called a dynamo by her colleagues. She served throughout France and was transferred to the hospital Llandovery Castle in early 1918 to effectuate a break from the intense workload she had face for almost 3 years.

III. The Fate of the U-Boat Captain Who Sunk the Llandovery Castle

Helmut Brümmer-Patzig (26 October 1890 – 11 March 1984) was the commander of U-Boat 86 who infamously sunk the hospital ship Llandovery Castle during World War I, but he also served from 1943 to 1945 as commander of a U-boat training group.

Despite international protocol and the Geneva Convention, he ignored the painted and lighted red crosses on the Llandovery Castle and sunk her with a torpedo. Under Patzig's command, crewmen were ordered to systematically ram and sink lifeboats carrying the few survivors, and then machine-gun any of the survivors in the water. In effect, he had murdered 234 persons. Fortunately, 24 people managed to disappear into the night in one lifeboat, and they lived to tell of the horrors perpetrated at the behest of Captain Patzig.

The story was extensively publicized throughout England, Canada and the U.S.A. during the remaining five months of the war. The victorious allies believed Patzig was a war criminal, but war fatigue made them decide to let the Germans prosecute him. That was a big mistake. Fearing retribution, he went into hiding for three years, but showed up in his birthplace, Danzig, in 1921. Danzig had been declared a free-city under the armistice agreement between Germany and the allies. Consequently, it was not under the jurisdiction of the German courts. It was not until 1931 that the free city status was revoked. By then, the Reichstag declared an amnesty for all war crimes committed in World War I. Patzig could now travel throughout Germany without fear of being tried for war crimes.

Patzig was a loyal supporter of Hitler and had many personal audiences with him. He served the Reich during World War II in a variety of places. His last placement was as a training officer. He drew a serviceman's pension and died at the age of 94 in 1984.

Unlike their Captain, the two watch officers of U-86 were tried in German Courts for war crimes and sentenced to four years each at hard labour. They served four months before they both escaped, never to be heard of again.

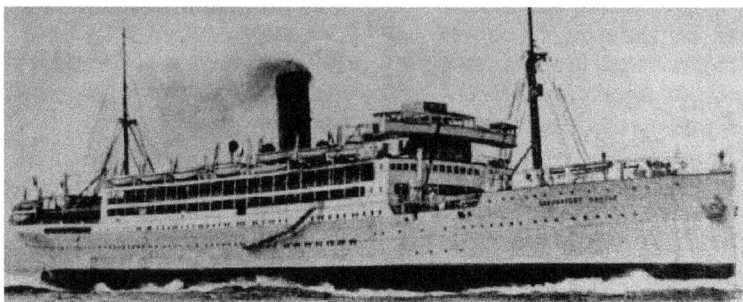

Llandovery Castle as it Appeared in 1912(before the war)[62]

IV. Nine Nurses Who Received the Military Medal for Bravery

Canadian women volunteering to serve as nurses flooded the army with applications. The offical tally of those killed during the World War I vary from 47 to 53, although the official count most often given is 47. The sacrifices made by these devoted nurses during World War I gave a needed boost to the women's suffrage movement in Canada. In fact, The Canadian Army nurses were among the first women in the entire world to win the right to vote as the Canadian Military Voters Act of 1917 extended the vote to women in military service. Although it sounds ridiculous that women were not allowed to vote, it was common practice almost everywhere in the world at the time; consequently, this act lent credibility to the women's suffrage movement.

Let us take a look at a few of the other Canadian nurses who served in World War I and were recipients of the Canadian Military Medal for Bravery.

---

[62] Retrieved from http://www.shipnostalgia.com/Passenger_Ship_ Disasters_-_6

Matron Edith Campbell

Born in 1871, Edith Campbell went to nursing school in Montreal, Quebec and rose to be a respected matron. In 1914, she volunteered for the Canadian Army Medical Corps at the age of 43 and was posted as a matron in the Étaples Hospital. She became well-known, not only in Canada, but in the United Kingdom, where she received the Military Medal for Bravery when she endured intense bombing and remained on duty the entire night to maintain discipline and efficiency to aid the wounded during a fierce battle.

When she arrived in England, she was appointed head matron, and along with physician Colonel Charles Wilson Gorrell, arranged with the Astor family to build a hospital on their huge estate in Cliveden. The first buildings were put on the tennis courts. Called the Duchess of Connaught Canadian Hospital, within a mere three weeks, Campbell and Correll had spearheaded the erection of a 550 bed hospital that would ultimately serve over 24,000 soldiers. It was primarily a recuperative hospital with sprawling lawns, recreational facilities and a state-of-the-art operating theatre. Having attained the rank of Captain, Edith Campbell, from all accounts was an imposing figure in her dress blue military uniform, and could always be seen in the wards urging her nurses to perform at peak efficiency.

The hospital was always spotlessly clean, and Campbell arranged for the men to have a vast array of recreational activities to help with their convalescence. Fresh flowers were placed on the men's lockers, and it seemed more like a home than a hospital. Above all, red tape was minimized so that things ran smoothly for the benefit of those being treated. Edith Campbell made sure that this place was a refuge from the horrors these men had faced on the front lines. She, herself, had been at Boulogne, France and received the Military Medal for Bravery for her heroic acts during the tumultuous bombing raids on the city. She had pleaded to stay at Boulogne, but was ordered back to the Duchess of Connaught Canadian Hospital to make sure things ran smoothly there.

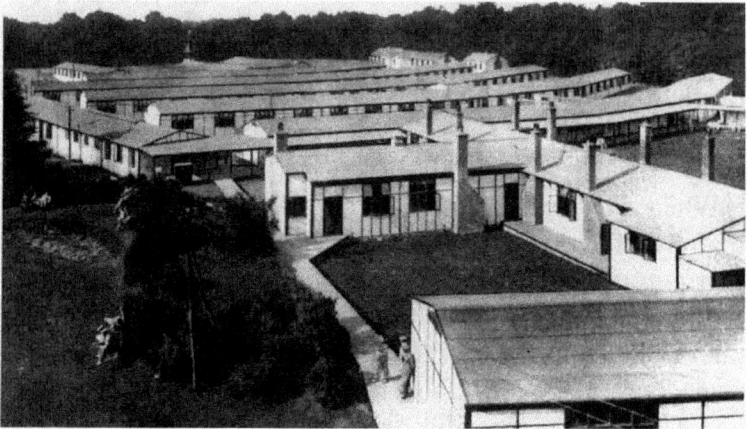

Duchess Connaught Canadian Hospital in Cliveden, UK (1915)[63]

Lenora Herrington

From Napanee, Ontario, Lenora received the Military Medal for Bravery for remaining on duty an entire night during heavy bombing and setting a personal example of courage by responsibly maintaining discipline and efficiency in an incredibly tense situation. While at an aid station near the front, she continued to fearlessly prep soldiers for surgery in an open area constantly subject to enemy bombardment and machine gun fire.

[63] Retrieved from http://www.crcmh.com/connaughtstage.jpg & www.greatwarproject

Lenora was encouraged to leave the area by several officers, but steadfastly requested to continue her duties. Her determination made them all acquiesce to the request, and the three officers jointly recommended her for the medal.

Janet Mary Williamson

When a bomb hit her ward, Janet was thrown several metres across the room. As mayhem ensued all about, she calmly got up and arranged for the evacuation of the patients as the ward burned. Supervising the removal of the patients at great personal risk, she insured their safety before leaving the ward herself. After the turmoil, Williamson ignored her own severely injured shoulder while continuing to aid her patients.

Meta Lodge and Eleanor Jean Thompson

It was a quiet evening on their ward, and Meta Lodge and Eleanor Thompson were setting at their desks when a horrendous explosion ripped through the ward and a beam fell across their table, penning them on the floor. Struggling to free themselves as their patients screamed in terror for aid, the two nurses finally managed, with the help of a patient, to free themselves. Noticing that the oil stoves had been overturned and flames were beginning to engulf the ward, they, along with the mobile patient, proceeded to douse the flames and then began to remove the patients. They continued to fearlessly go back into the rubble until each patient was removed.

Helen Elizabeth Hansen

Born in 1891, Helen became a nurse in 1913. Just as soon

as hostilities broke out, she was so anxious to enlist that she was the second one in line. Upon arrival in France, she was immediately dispatched to the western front hospitals, and proceeded to be recognized by her patients and superiors as a dedicated and competent nurse who always seemed to be on duty. Often, she would sleep in the ward, so she could be near her patients. That is why on the night her Étaples ward was bombed, she was present and able to extract patients from under debris and help with the evacuation. Her recommendation for the Canadian Military Medal for Bravery said in part, "Without trepidation or concern for her own safety, Nursing Sister Helen Elizabeth Hansen went above and beyond her duties to insure the safety and well-being of all the charges on her ward.

Mary Dow Lutwick

When the hospital was bombed from the air and ground, Mary Dow Lutwick got help for her patients and the nurses who had been injured by walking across an open bomb-swept ground alone in full view of the enemy aircraft and ground forces. She returned to the hospital and continued to work at the casualty clearing station while it was under fire from the enemy.

Beatrice McNair

The Germans attacked a bridge over the River Canche in Étaples, France in 1918. In the course of the German aerial bombing, both the Number 1 Canadian General Hospital and the Number 7 Canadian General Hospital were struck. Sixty-six Canadians were killed and 73 were wounded. Beatrice McNair and Helen Hansen (mentioned previously) were instrumental in maintaining discipline and caring for patients while the bombing continued.

Lottie Urquhart

When she enlisted in 1916, Lottie Urquhart volunteered for hospital ship duty, but when she found out that there was a shortage of nurses at front-line aid stations, she enthusiastically requested a duty assignment in France. Her citation for bravery reads, " For gallantry and devotion to duty during an enemy air raid, when four bombs fell on her ward. Regardless of danger she attended to the wounded. Her courage and devotion were an inspiring example to all."

These nine women were the first to receive combat medals, rather than service medals, and they are all a great testament to the devotion and professionalism of the Canadian nurses who served so gallantly and unselfishly in World War I.

Note:

Due to the scarcity of information available, the archives of the LONDON GAZETTE[64] were heavily relied upon for the information on the nine recipients of the Canadian Military Medal for Bravery. These women's devotion to serving their patients is a living testament for all nurses to look upon with pride.

V. The Brant Memorial and Dorothy Baldwin

Dorothy Yarwood Baldwin was 25 when she enlisted in 1917. She was born in Toronto and had been working as a nurse in Brantford, Ontario. She was assigned to the

---

[64] Retrieved from http://www.london-gazette.co.uk/search & www.greatwarproject.ca

Canadian Military Hospital in Doullens, France, and she was well known for her competence and devotion to patient welfare.

The hospital in Doullens was an ancient citadel from the 17th century and was cold, dark and dank. A riveting bombardment of the hospital on 19 May 1918 brought down almost the entire centre of the structure except for the exterior walls. Three nurses were killed instantly, along with 11 patients, two doctors and 16 other workers. Dorothy Baldwin, lying critically wounded as a fire raged through the complex, urged the rescuers to look after the patients before removing her from the debris. She was eventually evacuated, but died on 30 May 1918. Her final request was to be buried with her comrades. She is interred at the Bagneux Military Cemetery in Somme, France.

When the Brant War Memorial[65] was dedicated in 1933 in Brantford, Ontario, the first name listed was Dorothy Yarwood Baldwin.

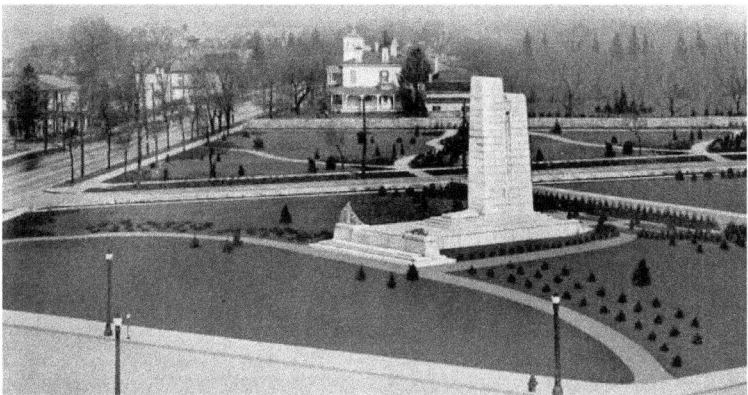

The Brant Memorial in Brantford, Ontario (Photo from 1933)

---

[65] Photo retrieved from http://www.brantwarmemorials.com

VI. Doing Their Duty

Prior to World War I, while some women attained a higher education and a few even managed to follow career paths reserved primarily for men, for the most part, women were expected to be primarily involved in domestic work related to the home. Before 1914, only a few countries had given the right to vote to women and apart from these countries (New Zealand and the Scandinavian nations), women were not even allowed to be involved in the political process. Yet, for many years, nursing had been a refuge for women who wanted more than just a home, a husband and children to look after. It was these women who were the vanguard of generations of women who would demand equality from governments that had made them second-class citizens.

Nursing was one of the only professions that afforded women the opportunity to directly contribute to the efforts on the battlefield. When Canadian nurses volunteered to serve during World War I, they were made commissioned officers before being sent overseas, a move that would grant them some authority in the ranks, so that enlisted patients and orderlies would have to comply with their direction. Canada was the first country in the world to grant women this privilege. At the beginning of the War, nurses were not dispatched to the casualty clearing stations near the front lines, where they would be exposed to shell fire. They were initially assigned to hospitals a relatively safe distance away from the front lines. As the war continued, however, nurses were assigned to casualty clearing stations and it was then that they began to come under direct fire from the enemy forces. Despite this, these brave women never wavered in their devotion and dedication to saving lives.

Nurses became increasingly respected, not only by the vast number of soldiers who made their way through aid stations and hospitals, but by the general staff officers who saw first hand their bravery and dedication to country and humanity. One general, after touring a Canadian hospital said, "the nurses work feverously to aid those suffering from the horrors of battle. They are our secret weapon that will eventually lead to the defeat of Germany."

Much of the credit for women getting the vote in Canada must go toward the nurses who served in World War I. The country's political leaders realized that it was unfair to ask women to serve when they did not have the right to vote, so the privilege was first extended to women in service, but fearing a backlash at home, the politicians wisely decided in 1917 to extend the vote to all females 18 or older.

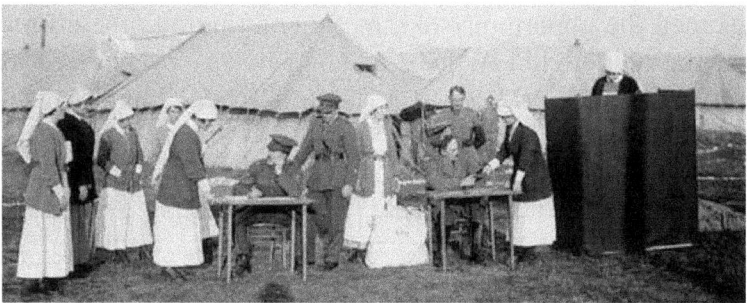

Nurses Lining Up to Vote in a Canadian Federal Election at an Aid Station On the Western Front in France (1917)[66]

Nurses were proclaimed war heroes by the Canadian soldiers and public. Their sacrifices and incredible dedication to duty permanently embedded in the minds of the people an abiding respect for them as competent

[66] Retrieved from http://en.wikipedia.org/wiki/Nursing

professionals. Unfortunately, there is little information available on these extraordinary women, who once the war was over, simply, for the most part, went back to serving in general hospitals all over Canada. Yet, their lives had been marked by war, and they and their profession would never be the same.

These women had witnessed first hand the horrors of war and the emotional effects it had on all who served. This recognition that a soldier can suffer just as much from psychological wounds as from physical wounds, made nurses strong advocates for mental health programmes that are now a vital component of the healthcare paradigm.

The price paid by these brave women is memorialized all across Canada in monuments to those who served, and those who died in World War I. As mentioned previously, the estimates of Canadian nurses killed in World War I generally varies between 47 and 53. The discrepancies might be because some actually made it back to Canada before dying as a result of injuries received while in Europe.

In 1928, a nurse, who had served in France, was introduced to a group of veterans at an Ottawa reunion of soldiers. Remembering the angels of mercy who had looked after them, the entire contingent of veterans stood and applauded. When asked after the convention what she thought of the ovation she received, her humble answer was simply, "they are the ones who should be applauded. It was our privilege to serve these men – it was our duty as Canadians."

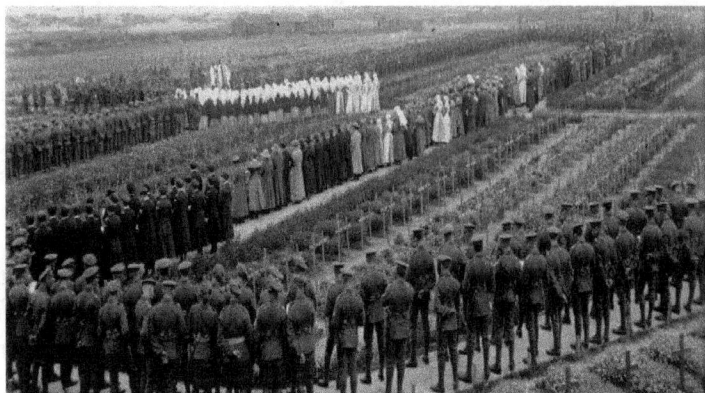

Nurses at Service for the Fallen on 4 August 1918 in
Étaples, France[67]

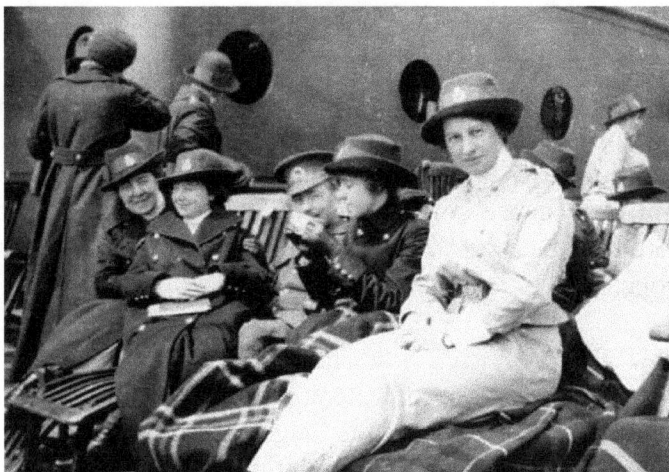

Nurses Were in a Jovial Mood as They Returned Home
From the War, But After a Few Weeks Leave, They Often
Pleaded to Be Sent Back As Soon As Possible [68]

[67] Retrieved from http://mp.natlib.govt.nz/detail/?id=81020&l=en
[68] Retrieved from http://data2.collectionscanada.gc.ca/ap/a/a202409.
jpg

This is the official roll of nurses listed as killed in World War I from Veterans Affairs Canada.[69] (This official document lists 49 deaths.)

1915
Matron JAGGARD, Jessie, Brown, 3rd Stationery Hospital
N/S MUNRO, Mary Frances E., 3rd Stationery Hospital

1916
N/S NOURSE, Grace E. Boyd, Canadian Army Military Corp (CAMC)
N/S ROSS, Elsie Gertrude, CAMC
N/S TUPPER, Addie Allen (Adruenna), Royal Red Cross (RRC) CAMC

1917
N/S GARBUTT, Sarah Ellen, (Ont Military Hospital)
N/S SPARKS, Letitia, (7 General Hospital)

1918
N/S ALPAUGH, Agnes, Estelle, CAMC
N/S ALPORT (Roberts), Jean, Ogilvie (4 General Hospital)
N/S BAKER, Miriam, Eastman (15 General Hospital)
N/S BALDWIN, Dorothy, Mary Yarwood (3 Stationery Hospital)
N/S BARTLETT, Bertha, (Newfoundland Voluntary Aid Detachment)
N/S CAMPBELL, Christina, (5 General Hospital)
N/S DAGG, Ainslie, St. Clair (15 General Hospital)
N/S DAVIS, Lena, A. (4 General Hospital)
N/S DOUGLAS, Carola Josephine, CAMC(H.S.)
N/S DUSSAULT, Alexina, CAMC(H.S.)

---

[69] Retrieved from
http://veterans.gc.ca/eng/history/other/Nursing/wardead

N/S FOLLETTE, Minnie Asenath, CAMC(H.S.)
N/S FORNERI, Agnes, Florien (8 General Hospital)
N/S FORTESCUE, Margaret, Jane, CAMC(H.S.)
Matron FRASER, Margaret, Marjory, CAMC(H.S.)
N/S FREDERICKSON, Christine, CAMC
N/S GALLAHER, Minnie Katherine, CAMC(H.S.)
N/S GREEN, Matilda Ethel, (7 General Hospital)
N/S HENNAN, Victoria, Belle (9 General Hospital)
N/S HUNT, Myrtle, Margaret CAMC
N/S JARVIS, Jessie Agnes, CAMC
N/S JENNER, Lenna Mae, CAMC
N/S KEALY, Ida Lilian, (1 General Hospital)
N/S LOWE, Margaret, (1 General Hospital)
N/S MCDIARMID, Jessie, Mabel (5 General Hospital)
N/S MACDONALD, Katherine, Maud (1 General
Hospital)
N/S MACEACHEN, Rebecca Helen, CAMC
N/S MCKAY, Evelyn, Verrall (3 General Hospital)
N/S MCKENZIE, Mary, Agnes, CAMC(H.S.)
N/S MCLEAN, Rena, R.R.C. (2 Stationery Hospital)
N/S MACPHERSON, Agnes, R.R.C. (3 Stationery
Hospital)
N/S MELLETT, Henrietta, (15 General Hospital)
N/S PRINGLE, Eden Lyal, (3 Stationery Hospital)
N/S ROGERS, Nellie Grace, CAMC
N/S ROSS, Ada Janet, (1 General Hospital)
N/S SAMPSON, Mary Belle, CAMC(H.S.)
N/S SARE, Gladys Irene, CAMC(H.S.)
N/S STAMERS, Anna Irene, CAMC(H.S.)
N/S TEMPLEMAN, Jean, CAMC(H.S.)
N/S TRUSDALE, Alice L., CAMC
N/S TWIST, Dorothy, Pearson (Canadian Military V.A.D.)
N/S WAKE, Gladys, Maude Mary, 1 General Hospital
N/S WHITELY, Anna Elizabeth, 10 Stationery Hospital

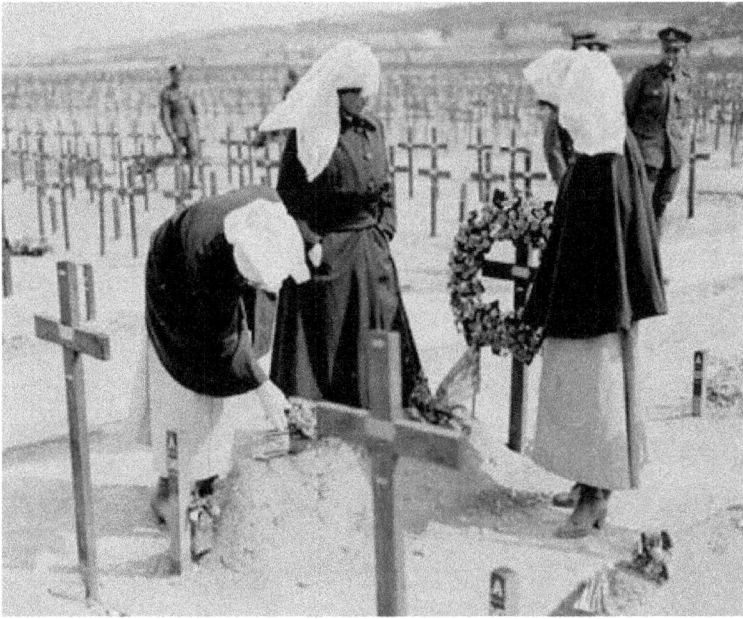

Nurses Honouring a Fallen Comrade in Étaples Cemetery
October 1918
(Photo from Canadian War Archives)

CHAPTER 10
AND THE WORST FRIEND AND ENEMY IS BUT DEATH

Although many nurses actually would, by necessity, wind up in the trenches to administer aid, most of the injured were brought back to the field hospitals by stretcher bearers or ambulances. There were thousands of women who valorously aided the injured, but one who simply called herself Violetta, was particularly adept at describing her life by the trenches. She left a diary that describes in simple terms some of the horrors faced by these brave women. In order to give our readers an idea of what it was like for these women, we offer a brief edited excerpt below:

I. Violetta by the Trenches

I was tired and weary but the next morning we went up to Radzivilow. It is the next station to Skiernevice, and there was very heavy fighting going on there when we went up. We were told we were going up on an armoured train, which sounded very thrilling, but when we got to the station we only found a quite ordinary carriage put on to the engine to take us up. The Russian battery was at that time at the south of the railway line, the German battery on the north of it, and we were in the centre of the sandwich. At Zyradow, these cannon sounded distant, but as we neared Radzivilow the guns were crashing away as they did at Lodz, and we prepared for a hot time. The station had been entirely wrecked and was simply in ruins, but the station-master's house near by was still intact, and we had orders to rig up a temporary dressing-station there.

Before we had time to unpack our dressings, a messenger arrived to tell us that the Germans had succeeded in enfilading a Russian trench close by, and that they were bringing fifty very badly wounded men to us almost at once. We had just time to start the sterilizer when the little carts began to arrive with some terribly wounded men. The machine guns had simply swept the trench from end to end. The worst of it was that some lived for hours when death would have been a more merciful release. Thank God we had plenty of morphine with us and could thus ease their terrible sufferings. One man had practically his whole face blown off, another had all his clothes and the flesh of his back all torn away. Another poor old fellow was brought in with nine wounds in the abdomen. He looked quite a patriarch with a long flowing beard, quite the oldest man I have seen in the Russian army. Poor Ivan, he had only just been called up to the front and this was his first battle. He was beautifully dressed, and so clean; his wife had prepared everything for him with such loving care, a warm knitted vest, and a white linen shirt most beautifully embroidered with scarlet in a intricate key-pattern. Ivan was almost more unhappy at his wife's beautiful work having to be cut than at his own terrible wounds. He was quite conscious and not in much pain, and did so long to live even a week or two longer, so that he might see his wife once again. But it was not to be, and he died early the next morning. He was one of the dearest old men one could ever meet, and so pathetically grateful for the very little we could do for him.

The shells were crashing over our heads and bursting everywhere, but we were too busy to heed them, as more and more men were brought to the dressing-station. It was an awful problem what to do with them: the house was small and we were using the two biggest rooms downstairs as operating and dressing-rooms. Straw was procured and laid on the floors of all the little rooms upstairs, and after each man's wounds were dressed, he was carried with difficulty up the narrow winding staircase and laid on the floor.

The day wore on and as it got dark we began to do the work under great difficulties, for there were no shutters or blinds to the upstairs windows, and we dared not have any light, even a candle there, as it would have brought down the German fire on us at once. So those poor men had to lie up there in the pitch dark, and one of us went round from time to time with a little electric torch. Downstairs we managed to darken the windows, but the dressings and operations had all to be done by candle-light.

The Germans were constantly sending up rockets of blue fire which illuminated the whole place, and we were afraid every moment they would find us out. Some of the shells had set houses near by on fire too, and the sky was lit up with a dull red glow. The carts bringing the men showed no lights, and they were lifted out in the dark when they arrived and laid in rows in the lobby till we had time to see to them. By nine o'clock that evening we had more than 300 men, and were thankful to see an ambulance train coming up the line to take them away. The stretcher bearers had a difficult job getting these poor men downstairs and carrying them to the train, which was quite dark too. However, the men were thankful themselves to get away. I think it was nerve-racking work for them, lying wounded in that little house with the shells bursting continually over it. You could see the anxiousness on their faces as they wondered whether they would live or die.

All night long the men were being brought in from the trenches. About four in the morning there was a little lull and some one made tea. I wonder what people back home would have thought if they had seen us at that meal. We had it in the stuffy dressing-room where we had been working without a stop for sixteen hours with tightly closed windows, and every smell that can be imagined pervading it, the floor covered with mud, blood and debris of dressings wherever there were not stretchers on which were men who had just been operated on. The meal of milk-less tea, black bread, and cheese, was spread on a sterilized towel on the operating-table, illuminated by two candles stuck in bottles. One exhausted nurse sat in the only chair, and the rest of us eased our weary feet by sitting on the edge of the dressing-boxes. Two dead soldiers lay at our feet, as it was not safe just at that moment to take them out and bury them. People would probably ask how we could eat under those conditions. I don't know how we could either, but we did and were thankful for it, for immediately afterward another rush of broken bodies began.

At eleven o'clock in the morning another ambulance train arrived and was quickly filled. By that time we had managed more than 750 patients through our hands, and they were still being brought in large numbers. The fighting must have been terrific, for the men were absolutely worn out when they arrived, and fell asleep at once from exhaustion, in spite of their wounds. Some of them must have been a long time in the trenches, for many were in a terribly vermin-infested condition. On one poor boy with a smashed leg you could have counted the insects by the millions. About ten minutes after his dressing was done, his white bandage was quite grey with the army of invaders that had collected on it from his other tattered garments.

Early that afternoon we got a message that another column was coming to relieve us, and that we were to return to Zyradow for a rest. We were very sorry to leave our little dressing-station, but rejoiced to hear that we were to go up again in two days' time to relieve this second column, and that we were to work alternately with them, forty-eight hours on, and then forty-eight hours off duty.

We had left Zyradow rather quiet, but when we came back we found the cannon going hard, both from the Radzivilow and the Goosof direction. It would have taken much more than cannon to keep us awake, however, and we lay down most gratefully on our stretchers in the empty room at the Red Cross Bureau and slept. A forty-eight hours spell is rather long for the staff, though probably there would have been great difficulty in changing the columns more often.

I woke up in the evening to hear the church bells ringing, and remembered that it was Christmas Eve, and that they were ringing for the Midnight Mass, so I got up quickly. The large church was packed with people, every one of the little side chapels was full and people were even sitting on the altar steps. There must have been three or four thousand people there, most of them, of course, the people of the place, but also soldiers, Red Cross workers and many refugees mostly from Lowice. Poor people, it was a sad Christmas for them, having lost so much already and not knowing from day to day if they would lose all, as at that time it was a question whether or not the Russian authorities would decide for strategic reasons to fall back once more.

And then twelve o'clock struck and the Mass began. Soon a young priest got up into the pulpit and gave them a little sermon. It was in Polish, but though I could not understand the words, I could tell from the people's faces what it was about. When he spoke of the horrors of war, the losses and the deaths and the suffering that had come to so many of them, one woman put her apron to her face and sobbed aloud in the tense silence. And in a moment, the whole congregation began sobbing and moaning and swaying themselves to and fro. The young priest stopped and left them alone a moment or two, and then began to speak in a low persuasive voice. I do not know what he said, but he gradually soothed them and made them happy. And then the organ began pealing out triumphantly, and while the guns crashed and thundered outside, the choir within sang of peace and goodwill to all men.

Christmas Day was a very mournful one for us, as we heard about the loss of our new and very best automobile, which had just been given as a magnificent present to the column a few days earlier. One of the boys was taking it to Warsaw from Skiernevice with some wounded officers, and it had broken down just outside the village. The mud was awful, and with the very greatest difficulty they managed to get it towed as far as Rawa, but had to finally abandon it to the Germans, though fortunately they got off safely themselves. It was a great blow to the column, as it was impossible to replace it, these big ambulance cars costing a great amount of money.

Food was very scarce at that time in Zyradow; there was hardly any meat or sugar, and no milk or eggs or white bread. One of us had brought a cake for Christmas from Warsaw weeks before, and it was partaken of on this melancholy occasion without enthusiasm. Even the punch made out of a teaspoonful of brandy from the bottom of a nurse's flask mixed with about a pint of water and two lumps of sugar failed to move us to any hilarity. Our menu did not vary in any particular from that usually provided at the restaurant, though we did feel we might have had a clean cloth for once.

We were very glad to go up to Radzivilow once more. Our former dressing-station had been abandoned as too dangerous for staff and patients, and the dressing and operating-room was now in a train about five-hubdred metres down the line from Radzivilow station. Our train was a permanency on the line, and we lived and worked in it, while twice a day an ambulance train came up, our wounded were transferred to it and taken away, and we filled up once more. We found things fairly quiet this time when we went up. The Germans had been making some very fierce attacks, trying to cross the river Rawka, and their losses must have been very heavy, but the Russians were merely holding their ground, and so there were comparatively few wounded on our side. This time we were able to divide up into shifts for the work, a luxury we were very seldom able to indulge in.

We had previously made great friends with a Siberian captain, and we found to our delight that he was living in a little hut close to our train. He asked me one day if I would like to go up to the positions with him and take some Christmas presents round to the men. Of course I was more than delighted, and as he was going up that night and I was not on duty, the general very kindly gave permission for me to go up too. In the end Colonel S. and one of the Russian Sisters accompanied us as well. The captain got a rough cart and horse to take us part of the way, and he and another man rode on horseback beside us. We started off about ten o'clock, a very bright moonlight night, so bright that we had to take off our brassards and anything that could have shown up white against the dark background of the woods. We drove as far as the pine-woods in which the Russian positions were, and left the cart and horses in charge of a Cossack while we were away. The general had intended that we should see the reserve trenches, but we had seen plenty of them before, and our captain meant that we should see all the fun that was going, so he took us right up to the front positions. We went through the wood silently in single file, taking care that if possible not even a twig should crackle under our feet, till we came to the very front trenches at the edge of the wood. We crouched down and watched for some time. Everything was brilliantly illuminated by the moonlight, and we had to be very careful not to show ourselves. A very fierce German attack was going on, and the bullets were pattering like hail on the trees all round us. We could see nothing for some time but the smoke of the rifles.

The Germans were only about a hundred yards away from us at this time, and we could see the river Rawka glittering below in the moonlight. What an absurd little river to have so much fighting about. That night it looked as if we could easily wade across it. The captain made a sign, and we crept with him along the edge of the wood, till we got to a Siberian officer's dug-out. At first we could not see anything, then we saw a hole between two bushes, and after slithering backwards down the hole, we got into a sort of cave that had been roofed in with poles and branches, and was absolutely invisible a few steps away. It was fearfully hot and frowzy with a little stove in the corner throwing out a great heat, and the men all began to smoke, which made it worse.

We stayed a while talking, and then crawled along to visit one of the men's dug-outs, a German bullet just missing us as we passed, and burying itself in a tree. There were six men already in the dug-out, so we did not attempt to get in, but gave them tobacco and matches, for which they were very grateful. These men had an "icon" or sacred picture hanging up inside their cave; the Russian soldiers on active service carry a regimental icon, and many carry them in their pockets too. One man had his life saved by his icon. He showed it to us; the bullet had gone just between the Mother and the Child, and was embedded in the wood.

It was all intensely interesting, and we left the positions with great reluctance, to return through the moonlit pine-woods till we reached our cart. We had indeed made a night of it, for it was five o'clock in the morning when we got back to the train once more, and both the doctor and I were on duty again at eight. But it was well worth losing a night's sleep to go up to the positions during a violent German attack. I wonder what the general would have said if he had known!

We finished our forty-eight hours' duty and returned once more to Zyradow. I was always loath to leave Radzivilow. The work there was splendid, and there more than anywhere else I have been to one feels the war as a high adventure. Yet, the adventure does not dull ones sense of the absolute horrors these men face 24 hours a day.

War would be the most glorious game in the world if it were not for the killing and wounding. In it one tastes the joy of comradeship to the full, the taking and giving, and helping and being helped in a way that would be impossible to conceive in the ordinary world. At Radzivilow, too, one could see the poetry of war, the zest of the frosty mornings, and the delight of the camp-fire at night, the warm, clean smell of the horses tethered everywhere, the keen hunger, the rough food sweetened by the sauce of danger, the riding out in high hope in the morning; even the returning wounded in the evening did not seem altogether such a bad thing out there. One has to die some time, and the Russian peasants esteem it a high honour to die for their "little

Mother" as they call their country. The vision of the high adventure is not often vouchsafed to one, but it is a good thing to have had it. It carries one through many a night in the shambles. In Belgium one's heart was wrung by the poignancy of it all, its littleness and defencelessness; in Lodz one could see nothing for the squalor and "frightfulness"; in other places the ruined villages, the flight of the dazed, terrified peasants show one of the darkest sides of war.

It was New Year's Eve when we returned to Zyradow, and found ourselves billeted in a new house where there was not only a bed each, but a bathroom and a bath. Imagine what that meant to people who had not undressed at night for more than three weeks.

Midnight struck as we were having supper, and we drank to the health of the New Year in many glasses of tea. What would the lifted veil of time disclose in this momentous year just opening for us?

It did not begin particularly auspiciously for me, for within the first few days of it I got a wound in the leg from a bit of shrapnel, was nearly killed by a bomb from a German plane, and caught a very bad chill and had to go to bed with pleurisy, all of which happenings gave me leisure to write this little account of my adventures.

The bomb from the tube was certainly the nearest escape I am ever likely to have in this world. I was walking over a piece of open ground, saw nothing, heard nothing, was dreaming in fact, when suddenly I heard a whirring overhead, and just above me was a German aeroplane. Before I had time to think, down came a bomb with a fearful explosion. I could not see anything for a minute, and then the smoke cleared away, and I was standing at the edge of a large hole. The bomb had fallen into a bed of soft mud, and exploded upwards. Some soldiers who were not very far off rushed to see if I was killed, and were very surprised to find that I was practically unhurt. A bomb thrown that same afternoon that exploded on the pavement killed and wounded nine people.

The wound was from a stray bit of shrapnel and was only a trifle, fortunately, and it soon healed. The pleurisy was a longer job and compelled me to go to bed for a fortnight. I was very miserable at being the only idle person I knew, till it occurred to me to spend my time in writing this little book, and a subsequent short holiday in Petrograd enabled me to finish it.

My enforced holiday is over now and I am on my way back to my beloved column once more - to the life on the open road - with its joys and sorrows, its comradeship, its pain and its inexplicable happiness, back once more to exchange the pen for the more ready weapon of the forceps.

And so I will leave this brief account of what I have seen in this great war. I know better than anyone can tell me what an imperfect sketch it is, but the history of the war will have to be studied from a great many different angles before a picture of it will be able to be presented in its true perspective, and it may be that this particular angle will be of some little interest to those who are interested in nursing work in different countries. Those who are workers themselves will forgive the roughness of the sketch, which was written during my illness in snatches and at odd times, on all sorts of stray pieces of paper and far from any books of reference; they will perhaps forget the imperfections in remembering that it has been written close to the turmoil of the battlefield, to the continual music of the cannon and the steady tramp of feet marching past my window. [70]

The last Canadian World War I veteran died in 2010 at the age of 110, so the oral history of the war is gone, but the contributions of nurses are memorialized through monuments, books, films and artefacts that attest to just how remarkable these women were. It is a legacy that all nurses should be immensely proud of, and they should all strive to live up to the examples set by these extraordinary women. The diaries of these women are a living testament to not only their bravery, but to the carnage that was wrought on the world and innocent people simply because human beings refused to settle their differences through negotiation and compromise rather than war.

II. *Dulce Et Decorum Est Pro Patria Mori (It is Sweet and Right)*

The following poem was written as a tribute to the nurses who braved the harshest of conditions to bring comfort to those who had suffered injuries on the fields of carnage.

THEY WERE AN INSPIRATION

Allons! After the great Companions, and to belong to them.
They too are on the road.
They are the swift and majestic, they are the greatest
women.
They know the universe itself as a road, as many roads,
As roads for travelling souls.
Camerados, I will give you my hand,

---

[70] Retrieved from http://www.ourstory.info/library/2-wwI/Thurstan/Journal.html

I give you my compassion more precious than money.
Will you give me yourselves, will you come travel with me?
Shall we stick by each other as long as we live?

—— *Anonymous soldier's tribute to the nurses[71]*

As time passes, we no longer can genuinely comprehend the tremendous sacrifices made by these women who served so valiantly, but we can still read about their exploits and how they brought honour, not only to a noble profession, but to Canada. Their devotion and sacrifice to eliminating the suffering of those who served in World War I, is generally an after-thought for most of us today, but the simple words of the men they served are illustrative of the high esteem in which they were held. Sometimes nothing more than a simple touch by a caring hand was enough to bring solace to those who suffered anguish and pain. Many of the soldiers tributes were anonymous, like the one below.

THE MERCIFUL

Because of you, we were glad and gay.
Remembering you, we will be brave.
We shall hail the advent of another dangerous day.
And meet the great adventure with a song.
You and your bluebird dress were filled with blood.
It was our blood and that of our comrades.
But through the horror, you gave us a smile
Oh, mercy, you show it to all us lads.

—— *Anonymous soldier's poem to his nurse (1915)[72]*

---

[71] Retrieved from http://www.ourstory.info/library/2-wwI/Thurstan/Journal.html
[72] Retrieved from http://www.outstory.info/library/2-ww1/journal

Many men were treated on the ambulance trains, which frequently would load up and pull out of the area in order to avoid bombardment while the nurses and surgeons were tending to patients. One soldier who was treated, left this on the table by his bed.

The Ambulance Train

The winter and the dark last long.
Grief grows and dawn delays.
Dear nurse, make our sword arm strong.
And lift high our gaze,
As our hearts weep.

Your lips speak words of hope,
So our promises we can keep.
We know our rest is a brief refrain,
Oh, the wonderful moments
with you on the ambulance train.

——— *Anonymous soldier on an ambulance train (1916)[73]*

Within this hell, nurses brought comfort, not just to those who suffered physically, but to those trapped in the throes of mental anguish as well. The nurses had to watch the terror within, when soldiers realized their legs, arms, speech or sight were gone. The horrors of deformed bodies were kept from the general public because it was not good for morale, but it could not be kept from those who saved their broken bodies. It was the nurses who had to help mend those broken in spirit as well as body, and give them the will to carry on. This stress caused great trauma among the nurses.

---

[73] Retrieved from http://www.War_Poems_Anonymous.com

One Nurse, Vera Brittain, scribed the following:

Sometimes in the middle of the night we have to turn people out of bed and make them sleep on the floor to make room for the more seriously ill ones who have come down from the line. We have heaps of gassed cases at present : there are 10 in this ward alone. I wish those people who write so glibly about this being a holy war, and the orators who talk so much about going on no matter how long the war lasts and what it may mean, could see a case - to say nothing of 10 cases of mustard gas in its early stages - could see the poor things all burnt and blistered all over with great suppurating blisters, with blind eyes - sometimes temporally, some times permanently - all sticky and stuck together, and always fighting for breath, their voices a whisper, saying their throats are closing and they know they are going to choke.

The strain is very, very great. The enemy is within shelling distance - refugee sisters crowding in with nerves all awry - bright moonlight, and aeroplanes carrying machine guns - ambulance trains jolting into the siding, all day, all night - gassed men on stretchers clawing the air - dying men reeking with mud and foul green stained bandages, shrieking and writhing in a grotesque travesty of manhood - dead men with fixed empty eyes and shiny yellow faces.[74]

Though not confirmed, it is assumed that she was the nurse who treated renowned World War I infantryman and poet, Wilfred Owen, twice. First when he was treated for mustard gas inhalation and secondly the day he was

---

[74] Retrieved from http://www.spartacusschoolnet.co.uk/FWWmustard. htm

brought in to an infirmary with a head wound that eventually proved fatal. Was she the inspiration for his most famous poem *Dulce et Decorum est* in 1917?

Dulce et Decorum est (1917)

Bent double, like old beggars under sacks,
Knock-kneed, coughing like hags, we cursed through sludge,
Till on the haunting flares we turned our backs,
And towards our distant rest began to trudge.
Men marched asleep. Many had lost their boots,
But limped on, blood-shod. All went lame, all blind;
Drunk with fatigue; deaf even to the hoots
Of gas-shells dropping softly behind.

Gas! Gas! Quick, boys! An ecstasy of fumbling,
Fitting the clumsy helmets just in time,
But someone still was yelling out and stumbling
And floundering like a man in fire or lime.
Dim through the misty panes and thick green light,
As under a green sea, I saw him drowning.
In all my dreams, before my helpless sight,
He plunges at me, guttering, choking, drowning.

If in some smothering dreams, you too could pace
Behind the wagon that we flung him in.
And watch the white eyes writhing in his face,
His hanging face, like a devil's sick of sin;
If you could hear, at every jolt, the blood
Come gargling from the froth-corrupted lungs,
Obscene as cancer, bitter as the cud
Of vile, incurable sores on innocent tongues,
My friend, you would not tell with such high zest
To children ardent for some desperate glory,

The old lie: *Dulce et decorum est Pro patria mori.* (It is sweet and right)

III. He Never Woke Again and We Kept Our Promise to Him

The Things They Carried is a collection of related stories by Tim O'Brien about a platoon of American soldiers in the Vietnam War, and how the things they carried with them into battle reflected who they were. Many times, it was left to the nurses who cared for them to gather their belongings when they were brought into aid stations. Nurses are often the last people with soldiers before they die. It is from these nurses that we have heard that the last word most often heard from dying soldiers is "Mama." How disheartening it must be to be by a bedside and know that a soldier, no matter how old, dies crying for his mother.

One of the authors of this book, Wayne Frye, also served in the military during the Vietnam War, and when conducting research for this book, he recalled a beautiful older nurse who tended to an injury he received while in basic training. The compassion and concern for his welfare exhibited by this woman was a profound influence on him and made him realize the impact one individual can have on the life of another. A few years ago, he adapted the recollections of a World War I nurse from the account of George Duhamel to pay tribute to all nurses like the one who took care of him. Duhamel knew that nurses were the core of healthcare, because it was they who spent the most time with patients. The soldiers of World War I saw nurses as a refuge from the inhumanity of war. The Canadian nurse in her Alice Blue Gown was a ray of sunshine in a world of darkness. They brought a smile to those who knew only privation in the trenches of despair through which they sloughed day after day. We proudly share here, an excerpt of Wayne Frye's retelling of Duhamel's story of the anguish faced by the angels of mercy during World War I. It is republished here in its short form.

AND RENA KEPT HER PROMISE TO HIM

The Rena Hamerhill Story by J. Wayne Frye

Canadian nursing sister Rena Hamerhill was stationed in the storied fields of Flanders at Passchendaele, Belgium. It was at this hospital that Colonel John McCrae, a surgeon, had written the most famous war poem ever penned. It was with that poem in mind that Rena surveyed the mangled and broken bodies that lay in the receiving area of the hospital and she could not help but recite the poem silently to herself.

In Flanders fields the poppies blow
Between the crosses, row on row,
That mark our place; and in the sky
The larks, still bravely singing, fly
Scarce heard amid the guns below.

We are the Dead. Short days ago
We lived, felt dawn, saw sunset glow,
Loved and were loved, and now we lie,
In Flanders fields.

Take up our quarrel with the foe:
To you from failing hands we throw
The torch; be yours to hold it high.
If ye break faith with us who die
We shall not sleep, though poppies grow
In Flanders fields.

Suddenly, as she regained her composure and moved about the receiving station to assess the conditions of her patients, a young corporal was brought in on a stretcher and placed on a gurney. Looking down at him sympathetically, she was about to learn that if modesty was banished from the face of the earth it would, no doubt, find refuge in the heart of this corporal.

He was covered in mud and tiny little pellets of stone from a shell that had probably burst overhead and sent out its deadly projectiles to sear the flesh of all within its treacherous path. His clothes were tattered and thread-bare. One of the aids had pulled his metal name tag out from around his neck and Rena saw that his last name was Morrison. He had a smooth, beard-free face and feigned a gentle smile as he said, "you'll have to excuse me, because it is hard for us to keep ourselves clean with all that mud in the trenches."

Somewhat amused at his concern about the way he looked, Rena smiled and said, "well, I wouldn't worry about your appearance, but we should be concerned about lice as they could infect your leg wound. Do you have any?"

Morrison, rather flush and uneasy, sheepishly replied, "I don't think so ma'am.

While Rena conversed with him, the orderly was cutting away what was left of his trousers. Looking down toward his legs, Rena immediately knew the young man had a major problem. The left leg had been completely mashed flat, and all that was left was a shattered mass of flesh. His boot dangled precariously to the side of the stretcher and the orderly was about to remove it. Morrison looked up at

Rena and said, "don't remove my boot. I am afraid my feet stink. I haven't had my boots off in nearly a week.

Rena placed her hand on his shoulder, smiling insipiently and said in her soft, melodic voice,, "don't worry about that, we have to remove it to give your leg the proper care that it needs. My dear Corporal Morrison, I have smelled the feet of many soldiers, and I have even had some princes as hospital patients, but I have never met any prince who is even worthy to take off your boots and wash your humble feet. You be quiet and let me do my job."

Then, Rena looked at his abdomen and realized that the leg wound was a minor problem to what she saw there. His fatigue jacket had been buttoned and tightly secured around his waist to help stop the sucking abdominal wound that had been stuffed with gauze. Turning to the doctor nearby she frantically shouted, "doctor."

Soon, the doctor arrived and with his forceps he lay hold carefully of a mass of bloody dressings, and drew them gently out of a gaping wound in the abdomen. A ray of sunshine filtered through the open shed door and lit him at his work, and the whole of the frail shed trembled as a bomb whizzed overhead.

"My mama is china-dealer," murmured Morrison to the doctor and Rena. "She has a big shop in Kent. Save me, and you shall see. I'll give you a fine piece of china. You can save me can't you? My mama will be so hurt if I don't make it back. I am not her only son, but I am her youngest, her baby. It would be so hard on her, if I don't come back."

The surgery was franticly done as time was of the essence;

the forceps glittered, and the rays of sunshine seemed to tremble under the cannonade, as did the floor, the walls, the light roof, the whole earth, the whole universe, drunk with fatigue and anguish.

Suddenly, from the depths of space, a whirring sound arose, swelled, ascended high above the shed, and the shell burst a few feet away, with a thud that shattered the dense air of the shed. The thin walls seemed to quiver under the pressure of the resounding reverberation. The doctor made a slight movement of his head, but never took his eyes off Morrison. Rena swabbed his forehead gently, looked down at Morrison, smiled and took his right hand in hers.

Then Morrison said in a quiet, quivering voice, "don't take any notice of those small things, they don't do any harm. Only save me, and I will give you a beautiful piece of china or earthenware, whichever you like. My mama will let you pick out whatever you want."

Rena thought to herself, if only it were that simple. If only you could barter for life with a piece of china. She wanted to cry, but she fought back the tears, because she did not want to alarm Morrison.

Rena knew that the situation was tenuous at best. His leg wound was not fatal. The pellets imbedded here and there in his soft, boyish flesh were minor, but the huge abdominal wound was sucking the life out of this young man who desperately wanted to live not for himself, but to save his mother pain.

With his livid lips, no longer distinguishable from the rest of his face, and the immense black pupils of his eyes, Morrison showed a countenance irradiated by a steadfast soul, which would not give in until the last moment. Morrison contemplated the ravages of his body almost severely, and without illusion, and watching the surgeon as he scrubbed his hands, almost in disgust at his obvious failure, he said in a grave voice, "tell my mama that my last thoughts were of her."

He uttered, "tell her, please tell her."

It was not a veiled question, for, without a moment's hesitation, he looked deep into Rena's eyes and managed a faint smile. His boyish face was not the face of one who could be deceived by soft words and consoling phrases. Rena, still holding his hand, as other patients were crying out in pain, could not turn away. The surgeon's eyes grew dim as he realized that he was about to lose another patient in the endless of sea of injured that flowed like a river through the hell that was known as the western front.

Meanwhile Rena, knowing that Morrison was ready to accept his fate, whispered softly, "we will not fail to do so, my dear friend. Your mother will know your last thoughts were of her."

The patient's eyelids fluttered and gently closed, as he fell into a deep slumber. He never woke again, and Rena kept her promise to him.[75]

---

[75] Reprinted from the 2003 Interpretational Analysis of Rena Hamerhill's Journal: A Nurse's Inspiration in Flanders Fields – Shortened Version by J. Wayne Frye

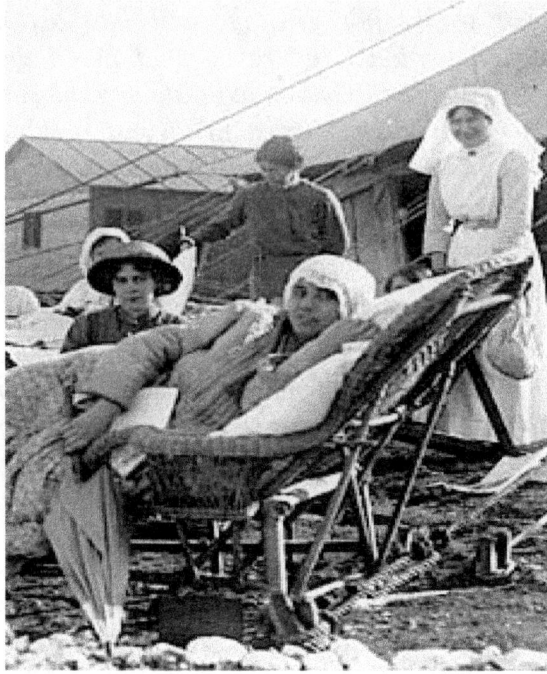

Passchendaele Hospital #4 Where the Nurses Often Slept Outside to Make More Room for Patients Because of Over-crowding in the Wards[76]

IV. Rendition on a Soldier's Sacrifice as an Illustration of the Subtle Impact of Nurses on the Mental Health of Patients

A simple diary entry was often meant by a nurse as nothing more than a record of her experiences, but today their diaries also serve as a testament, not only to the bravery of soldiers, but to the healing power of nurses who offer more than relief from physical pain. They are vital to the emotional welfare of patients as well. A kind word, a

[76] Retrieved from http://www.trove.nla.gov.au/list?id=1498

little encouragement or a caring touch can often be a vital adjunct to the physical healing process. Our below short story, based on a nurse's diary is illustrative of the healing power of a smile, compassion and a few kind words.

MY HERO

We had all the windows opened. From their beds, the wounded could see through the dancing waves of heat, the heights of Berru and Nogent l'Abbesse, the towers of the Cathedral, still crouching like a dying lion, and the chalky lines of the trenches intersecting the landscape.

A kind of torpor seemed to hang over the battle-field. Sometimes, a perpendicular column of smoke rose up, in the motionless distance, and the detonation reached us a little while afterwards.

It was one of the fine days of summer 1915, one of those days when the supreme indifference of nature makes one feel the burden of war more cruelly, when the beauty of the sky seems to proclaim its remoteness from the anguish of the human heart.

We had just finished the morning rounds when a rickety, squeaky ambulance pulled up to the entrance. Peering out of the ambulance at me in my Alice Blue Gown, the soldier looked me up and down, as if he was trying to undress me with his eyes. Yet, I was not offended as I thought how wonderful that a man could still have thoughts of passion in all this turmoil.

I moved closer to the vehicle as the driver got out and opened the back doors. Turning to me, he said, "I have three critically wounded men."

Then, from inside the vehicle came a low, excited, pleading voice that reverberated with extreme fear. "I am severely wounded, please – please help me."

He was not a man, just a mere boy whom I later found out he was 18, but he appeared no more than 14 or 15.

"Oh, I am in such pain," he said.

He held tightly onto the stretcher with his right hand while reaching out for me with his left. As he was carried into the prep ward, I reached down and took his left hand. He squeezed hard like a little boy pleading with his mother to not let go of him.

Looking about the room, now filled with agonizing cries from the other wounded who had been brought in, he appeared astonished and confused as a grey pallor seemed to overcome him. I reached down and covered his face with a chloroform-filled gauze and he fell at once into a deep, peaceful sleep.

The doctor came over, looked down at both his shattered legs and said, "The right leg. The right leg. Oh my. It can't be saved."

The burden of the experience, like so many others, weighed heavily upon me as I contemplated his waking after the amputation and seeing that he no longer had his right leg.

Private Comstock lay in bed for hours after the amputation, catching his breaths with difficulty and occasionally sobbing in his unconscious state. Suddenly he woke up, looked about languidly, and gazed at the bottle of serum, the needles in his arm and all the apparatuses used to revive his fluttering heart. His parched lips seemed to be begging for a drink that I could not give, and his eyes fixed on mine almost pleading for the release offered by death.

His head turned toward the narrow doorway bordered by sandbags and he sighed as he drifted off, lost in that twilight between life and death. Which would he choose?

Hour after hour passed, as I tended to his needs, he rarely uttered a word, only looked forlornly at me with tears in his eyes. Yet, death, which had sought him so boldly, seemed to retire, yielding ground by degrees, until it was finally halted. However, his mental state seemed to constantly be in peril, as he avoided looking down where his right leg should have been. I could not let him feel defeated.

We had to help him fight for the portion of his soul death had chosen. Finally, when he looked down where his leg should have been, he seemed unsure of whether he should utter thanks or rail against us for taking his leg.

As soon as he could speak, he said to me, "you have cut off my leg."

I struggled for words of solace that would not come, as his eyes filled and his head sank low into the fluffy, while pillow and tears trickled down his cheeks. All I could do was reach over, take his hand and squeeze it in mine.

He drifted off into a peaceful slumber still sobbing. The next day, as I redid his dressings, he was obviously in a great deal of pain. He looked down at his stub that were oozing pus and blood, trembling as he said "it looks horrible doesn't it?"

I replied with a faint smile pursing my lips, "it looks much worse than it is. You are going to be fine."

Looking down at his narrow chest, his thin face and his boyish forehead with one serious furrow in it, I did not know how to show him my respect and affection. I looked out the window and the rays of the morning sun seemed to bounce about his head, almost giving him an angelic glow. Yet, I knew all was not well. His left leg was now seriously infected near the lower thigh. I laboriously contemplated how we could tell him that we might have to remove his other leg.

I thought to myself that a man does not die of pain, or Private Comstock would already be dead. I watched as he valiantly fought against the desire to scream. His eyes were desperately pleading for relief as he endured unimaginable agony. I called on the doctor for help, as I encouraged him to scream if he wanted. Yet, he struggled to subdue his desire to cry-out. Finally, as the doctor, I and three other nurses held him, he finally let all his anguish out as his screams reverberated throughout the ward.

Injecting him with morphine, the agony continued for what seemed like hours as we frantically restrained his seething, writhing body that fought furiously for release from the agony. Finally, the morphine's power surged through his body into the brain, fooling it into believing the pain had subsided.

The doctor turned to me after he looked at his badly infected left leg and said, "he must make another sacrifice."

Comstock was not asleep, and the doctor suddenly realized that he should not have made the statement to me in front of him.

Comstock understood what had to be done to save him. He stopped weeping. He had the leaguered look of a man who was rowing against the tide. I stared down at him as he said, "I would rather die than be half a man. Please, please help me to die."

Within a few minutes he drifted unwilling off to sleep. Overcome with intense emotion, I asked permission to go outside for some fresh air and a respite from the cries of agony in the ward. I strolled through the mud street, head down, oblivious to everything around me as I thought over and over what he said. "I would rather die than be half a man."

I find myself asking whether we should grant his request. Would it not be more merciful to let him go? Then a voice in my head said, "no, he will never be half a man. With no legs, he will be more than most men whose legs are whole."

It was then that I realized my mission as a nurse was more than repairing bodies. The body was an adjunct of the soul. The soul of man was capable of soaring beyond the restraints imposed by the body. I had to reach the souls of those for whom I cared.

That evening, the surgeon came by and talked with Comstock. Yet he was determined not to have his leg amputated. The surgeon signalled for me to follow him out of the ward. In the hallway, he said, "you must convince him." Yet, I realized that I, myself, would feel the same way. How can I convince someone to do something I would not do."

Lounging in a chair, relishing the warm, cloudless summer evening, I felt ashamed that I had contemplated agreement with Comstock. Yet, I asked myself what could I offer him in exchange for what I was going to ask of him. Where could I find the words that would induce a man to live?

That morning, I laboriously cleaned his infected left leg. He secretly concluded that this would perhaps make the amputation unnecessary, and it greatly pained me to see his joy. I knew that I could not let him continue with the illusion.

The inner struggle began again, as I understood the situation was desperate and that we were under the restraints of time. Every hour of delay made the situation more dire. A day or two more and there would be no choice open to him, only a painful, agonizing death.

His refrain never ceased, "I am not afraid, but I would rather die."

How could I talk to him as an advocate for life? Who gave me the right? Who gave me eloquence? Anyway, I could give him no guarantees that the operation would save his life. And how could I tell him of a bright future that lay ahead without his legs? I asked myself how would I feel were I in that bed, missing one leg and facing the possibility of losing another? Yet, I felt compelled to assert for life over death. Was that not my purpose as a nurse – to affirm life?

I talked to him periodically while on duty, and, when off duty, I sat by his bedside, reading to him and discussing his life. He said, "I live with my mother. I cannot expect her to take care of me the rest of my life. What will I do when she dies? There is no work for cripples."

I replied, "your mother would never see you as a cripple. You are her son. Your country would not see you as a cripple, but as a hero who stood by her when she needed you."

I saw the germination of deep thoughts take hold as he stared off into space. It was then that I encouraged him to let me get him up and push him outside in a wheelchair, so that he could enjoy the cool night air as a respite from the stuffy ward.

We sat at the edge of the terrace. I reached over and took his feeble wrist so I could check his pulse. It was beating furiously. The night sky was penetrated with streamers as both armies were lighting the battlefields nearby. The rat-a-tat-tat of gunfire seemed to be so faint that it almost added a rhythmic beauty to the night. Rockets rose above the nearby hills and fell slowly with their customary whiz, lighting the countryside with an amber glow. Through it all, Comstock remained contemplative. I placed my left hand on his right shoulder as I stood by his side. I did not have to say a word to him, because he knew that I had a deep simpatico for him and the turmoil that was raging within his soul.

Then, he whispered "I don't know. I don't know."

I knew he was ready. He said he didn't know, but he did. By simply not knowing, he was now ready to embrace life.

On the next morning, before the operation, he asked me to wheel him outside once again. He looked all about, as if he wanted to witness the joy of life just in case he did not wake up from the anaesthetic. We shared a smile and he said, "I hope it is not too late."

I pushed him back toward the ward and whispered, "it will be alright." Yet, I knew that it might not. His condition was precarious, and his hesitation could have allowed the infection to spread.

He begged the surgeon to allow me to assist, and I was graciously afforded the opportunity to standby as he lay on the operating table. We cut through flesh and bones. The surgeon amputated a bit higher than was necessary, because he wanted to make sure he got all the infection.

I followed the orderly as he rolled Comstock back to the ward, and I helped to gently remove him from the gurney and place him in his bed. I could not help but notice how light he was with both his legs gone. I continued with my duties, but checked back on him constantly, waiting for him to awaken. Finally, when off duty, I sat by his bed, so that when he finally awakened from his drug induced slumber that a familiar face would be there to greet him.

When he blinked his eyes and looked up at me, he did not say a word. Nor did I. Simply reaching out with my hand, I patted his right arm. He gave me a forced smile, closed his eyes and returned to slumber.

As the days passed, I watched Comstock's strength gradually grow, and he seemed less dependent on me as an emotional crutch. Still, there was always a certain glow about him every time he saw me. I began to feel that he was helping me as much as I was helping him. I could see the admiration and appreciation in his interaction with me.

And, his compassion for other patients was apparent as he was constantly giving them encouragement and trying to let them know that things might look bad, but they would get better.

He became an incredibly sensitive person. He was touched by all that he saw around him, and would often look at me after discussing the agony others were going through and say, "I don't have it so bad."

When he spoke of his own case, he made light of his own misfortune. I began to watch him with admiration, and he seemed to always be encouraging me to help others who needed a boost in their spirits. He would say, "you can lift his spirits, like you did mine. I know you can."

He became so self-sufficient that I found myself not needing to spend as much time with him, as there were others who needed me more. Yet, I always made it a point to tell him good-bye when my shift would end, and, on occasion, would come back while off duty to read to him or share a snack. He seemed ever so grateful that I took the time to do so.

I was always careful to never call attention to Comstock's missing limbs, but one day when I was removing the dressing, he suddenly reached back with both hands and threw himself on his shoulders, holding his stumps up in the air. As they pointed toward the ceiling he said, "put some torpedoes on them and I could blow the roof off."

The whole ward burst out in laughter, me included. Was he finally over the crisis of self-doubt. I thought so, but would find that there was one more hurdle he had to overcome.

As I was attending to my duties in the ward the next morning, several soldiers were talking of love, marriage and a home. I glanced over toward Comstock and saw something I had not seen for weeks. He seemed despondent and uninterested in conversing with the others who had all come to admire him for his positive attitude. In fact, Comstock had become quiet the hero among the others, as they saw him as the one who faced the greatest adversity and had overcome it.

I stood by his beside and whispered, "aren't you interested in the conversation?"

He frowned and replied, "I will never have a wife or children now."

Then I told him something I knew about women and their penchant for love. I explained that a man did not need legs to procure the love of a woman. He needed honesty, self-assurance, a kind nature, a sense of humour, and above all, a deep commitment to the one he loved.

He appeared a bit perplexed and said, "I am worried about something else you do when you are married. I can't talk to you about it."

I gave him my somewhat mischievous, devilish smile and said, "I think I know what you mean, and I assure you that part of you was not amputated. Even if it had been amputated, for most women, love goes far beyond the mere physical."

We both laughed, but his consternation was only mildly assuaged. He looked down at his missing legs forlornly and then back up at me. I knew that he was thinking his lack of legs would be a problem in performing what he considered his duties as a husband."

Maintaining my decorum, I simply said with confidence, "when it comes to that, two people in love can overcome any obstacle."

He confidently smiled at me and replied somewhat sheepishly, "know anybody who wants to help me practice?"

I did not say a word in reply. I simply got up, smiled and walked down the ward. As I exited, I could hear Comstock conversing with the others, and knew that there were many women who would find him appealing, even without legs. Now, he knew that ,too.

Comstock received a visit from a general who awarded him two medals for bravery. Afterward, I was explaining to him that he would be able to walk with artificial legs. He looked at me and said, "hey, I was pretty short before. Now I can be as tall as I want."

We laughed together, and then he asked to go outside. All the wheelchairs were in use, so I told him I would have to carry him. He looked all about, finally gazing down where his legs should have been, and he laughingly said, "well, I only weigh half as much as I used to, so go ahead."

Not being a small girl, I never hesitated. I just reached down, lifted him from the bed and proceeded out of the ward, carrying him like a baby. Comstock and the rest of the ward were ecstatic with laughter. Walking onto the terrace, I carefully placed him in a chair. I was actually pleased with myself.

He had the two medals in his hand. He blushed a bit as he said, "I don't really deserve these. I was just doing my duty. Many others were killed on both sides. The ones who died are the real heroes, they gave much more of themselves than I did."

Searching for a reply that would justify the medals, I said, "we all are just doing our duty, but some of us do it better than others. Do not disparage yourself, because you lived and others died. That is fate, over which we have no control."

I then recited what the general, when presenting the medals, had said about his courage that had saved the lives of so many the day he was injured. But it was not enough to satisfy his disdain for being called a hero. He said, "you deserve them more than I. You save so many, while I only saved a few."

I must admit to a sense of pride when I realized that he appreciated my efforts. All I could say was, "I am just doing my duty." Then, we smiled at each other, eased back and sat quietly enjoying the moment in sublime pleasure and mutual respect.

The day came when we had to part. The war went on, and the carnage continued to flood the hospital with more broken bodies and wounded spirits. There would be many more Comstocks. Some would, like him, rise to the occasion and emerge victorious, and others would succumb to despair and hopelessness. All I could do was hope for the best and continue to try and heal those broken in body and spirit. Throughout the years, I always remembered Comstock and wondered how he was doing. I knew he lived in Manitoba, but I never heard from him until one day in 1961 when a small package arrived at my home on Prince Edward Island.

Opening it with my now frail, aged hands, there was a newspaper clipping. It was an obituary. I read with much trepidation about the death of a World War I veteran named Comstock. There was a letter from his wife that read, "my dear husband, on his deathbed, asked me to see that you received the two items enclosed. I apologize for waiting six months to forward this, but it was difficult finding you after all these years. Finally, I realized that the Veterans Affairs Office would probably know your location. I cannot thank you enough for all you did for him. He spoke of you often. He also wanted me to tell you that three of our five grandchildren are nurses. He had a grand and wonderful life, and he always said that you were, in a large part, responsible for that."

The items were wrapped in linen, and as I delicately removed it, tears began to swell in my eyes, because I knew what was there even before gazing upon them, Comstock's two medals for bravery. There was a small white note wedged between the two medals.

I looked at them, caressed them gently, and thought back on those days with him in the hospital. Those days long ago, when in my fleeting youth, I was in awe of the bravery of so many men who sacrificed all they could give to a grand and noble cause. Yet, Comstock always stood out among them.

Opening the note gently, as if it was the most prized possession I owned, the tears began to cascade down my cheeks. There were only two words in bold, big letters - **MY HERO**.

V. Often No Victory Over the Final Enemy, But The Will To Battle It With Great Tenacity

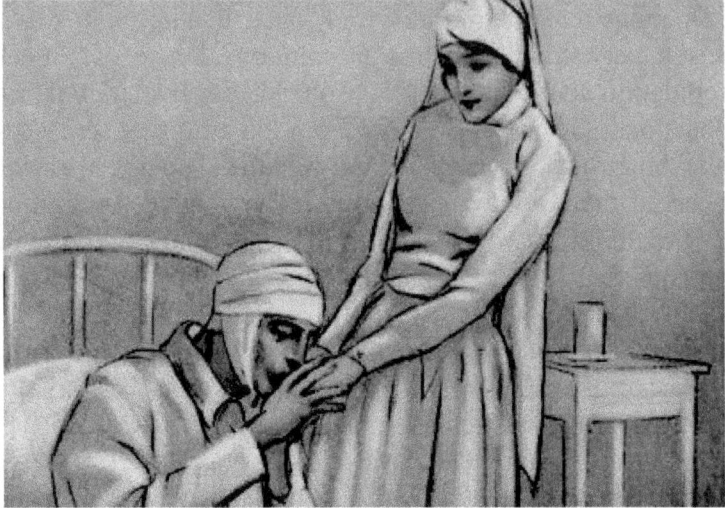

The Soldiers Idolized the Nurses Who Cared for Them as Depicted in the Above Illustration from World War I [77]

No amount of training could have properly prepared the nurses for the horrors they faced in World War I. The artillery used by the armies of the time was designed to inflict massive injuries to bodies. The wounds were more vicious and horrific than in any previous war. Then, there was the use of some of the most insidious weapons ever devised, like poisonous gas and blistering agents that were packed into artillery shells and exploded over soldiers to inflict horrendous agony through a slow, methodical, terrifying death. One can only barely comprehend the horrors faced by these women who had to deal with this on a daily basis.

------

[77] Retrieved from http://www.nursepostcard.com/gallery.html

Nurses were usually thrown into this hell with no psychological preparation for what they would witness. Not only were they treating wounds they had never before seen, or even in some cases, contemplated, but they were exposed to enemy fire in hospitals and aid-stations that were once considered safe-havens from combat.

The below excerpt from a nurse's diary is indicative of the compassion, mercy and respect showed to those they served.

Would that I could do more than thank the dear friends who made my life for four years so happy and contented; who never made me feel by word or act, that my self-imposed occupation was otherwise than one which would ennoble any woman. If ever any aid was given through my own exertions, or any labour rendered effective by me for the good of the my country, if any sick soldier ever benefited by my happy face or pleasant smiles at his bedside, or death was ever soothed by gentle words of hope and tender care, such results were only owing to the cheering encouragement I received from them. They were gentlemen in every sense of the word, and though they might not have remembered that "noblesse oblige," they felt and acted up to the motto in every act of their lives. My only wish was to live and die among them, growing each day better from contact with their gentle, kindly sympathies and heroic hearts.[78]

There are no statistics available, but there were, no doubt, numbers of these women who came back from the war with what would now be diagnosed as post-traumatic stress disorder. It is almost unimaginable what these brave

---

[78] Retrieved from http://www.civilwarhome.com/civilwarnurses.htm

women went through, but through it all, they served with great dignity and pride.

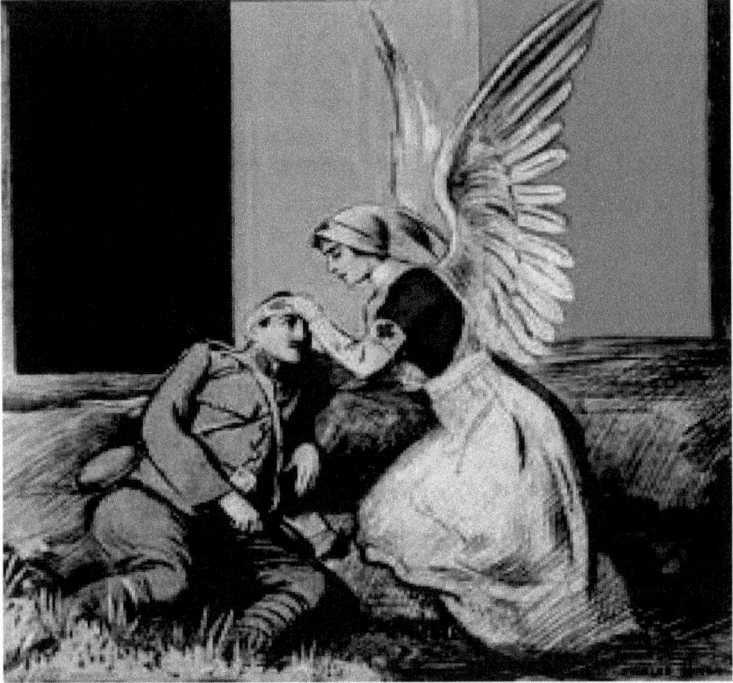

Above is From a World War I Post-Card Depicting the High Esteem In Which Nurses Were Held by Soldiers[79]

Most of the nurses were ill-prepared through their studies to deal with the psychological damage inflicted on the soldiers, but they valiantly offered encouragement and compassion that lifted countless thousands from the doldrums of despair. They always thought of death as their enemy, as exemplified by the following scroll that hung at the entrance to a field hospital in Flanders. It is assumed to be written by a nurse.

---

[79] Retrieved from http://www.nursepostcard.com/gallery.html

Naught broken save this body, lost but breath.
Nothing to shake the laughing heart's long peace there,
But only agony, and that has ending;
And the worst friend and enemy is but Death.[80]

---

[80] Retrieved from http://www.gutenberg.org/files/18910/18910-h/18910-h.htm

CHAPTER 11
THEY SHOULD BE AT THE FRONT OF THE LINE

To better understand what the war was like for the nurses, let's take a look at one of the most ferocious bombardments in the war that occurred in Lodz, Poland. The valour of the nurses during this bombardment was attested to by hundreds who witnessed their heroic endeavours to serve those in need. The retelling of the story of Lodz follows on the next page.

World War I Official Military Map of Lodz on the Polish Front[81]

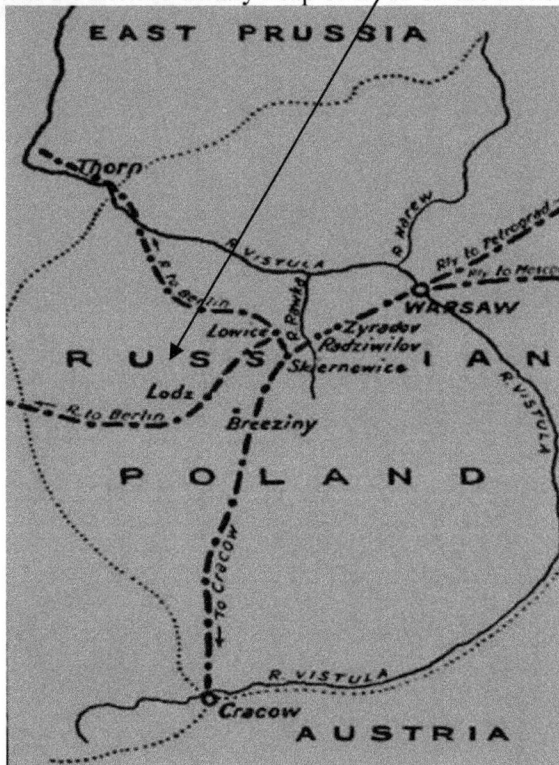

---

[81] Retrieved from http://www.gutenberg.org/files/17587/17587-h/17587-h.htm#Page_93

VIOLETTA AT LODZ

World War I saw the introduction of something called the Flying Column, which was a term applied to the mobile medical service that was supposed to go anywhere at anytime at any hour of the day. The medical column that was sent to Lodz consisted of five automobiles that conveyed doctors, nurses, medical staff and all equipment to the place where they were to work, and then they engaged in fetching in wounded, and taking them on to the field hospital or ambulance train. They had to unload cotton-wool covers, bandages, dressings, anaesthetics, field sterilizers, operating-theatre equipment and a certain amount of stores, such as soap, candles, benzene and tinned food, all while bombs were going off nearby. The Russian front changed so much more rapidly than the Anglo-French front, where progress was reckoned in metres, that these mobile columns were a great feature of ambulance work there. The front changed many kilometres in a week sometimes, so that units that could move anywhere at an hour's notice were very useful. The big base hospitals could not quite fulfill the same need on such a rapidly changing front.

The nurses were ferried to Lodz by convoy and the roads were villainously bad anyway, and the Germans, though their retreat had been hasty, had taken time to destroy the roads and bridges as they left. Another thing that delayed the convoy was the enormous reinforcements of troops going up from Warsaw to the front. As the convoy drew nearer to Lodz it was typical to see a good many dead horses lying by the roadside, mostly killed by shell-fire. The shells had made great holes in the road, and the last part of the journey was like a ride on a rough roller coaster, only in slow motion. It began to get dark as the medical convoy came to Breeziny, where a large number of Russian batteries were stationed. It was very jolly there, these large camps of men and horses having their supper by the light of a crackling, roaring camp-fire, with only the distant rumble of the guns to remind them that they were at war. Yet, one sensed that the jolliness was only a transitory way of forgetting the agony and misery they faced in the trenches each day.

Lodz was a large cotton manufacturing town, sometimes called the Manchester of Poland, but at this time all the factories were closed, and many destroyed by the intensive bombing. It had never been a very festive place at the best of times; but now it looked even more squalid and grimy, and the large bulk of its population was made up of the most abject people one could imagine as they endured the constant bombardment.

The column had to make a long detour and get into the town by an unfrequented country road. The medical corps was put down at a large building which they were told was the military hospital. Upon arrival the group noticed a resident surgeon and a student surgeon were working hard in the operating-room, and they hastily put on clean overalls and joined them. They all looked absolutely worn out, and the doctor dropped asleep between each case; but fresh wounded were being brought in every minute and there was no one else to help. Lodz was one big hospital. They heard that there were more than 18,000 wounded there, and the medical staff was simply overwhelmed. Every building of any size had been turned into a hospital, and almost all the medical supplies had been exhausted. Thus begins another scenario by Violetta, the same nurse who had eloquently recorded her experiences by the trenches.

The Bombardment of Lodz

The building we were in had been a day-school, and the top floor was made up of large airy schoolrooms that were quite suitable for wards. But the shelling recommenced so violently that the wounded all had to be moved down to the ground floor and into the cellars. The place was an absolute inferno. I could never have imagined anything worse. It was fearfully cold, and the hospital was not heated at all, for there was no wood or coal in Lodz, and for the same reason the gas-jets gave out only the faintest glimmer of light. There was no clean linen, and the poor fellows were lying there still in their vermin-infested, blood-soaked shirts, shivering with cold, as we had only one small blanket each for them. They were lucky if they had a bed at all, for many were lying with only a little straw between them and the cold stone floor. There were no basins or towels or anything to wash up with, and no real plumbing, so the men were placing bed pans by their side, waiting for staff to dispose of them. In the largest ward where there were seventy or eighty men lying, there was a lavatory adjoining which had gotten blocked up, and a thin stream of dirty water trickled under the door and meandered in little rivulets all over the room. The smell was awful, as some of the men had been there already several days without having had their dressings done. We were appalled by the sanitary conditions, but what could we do?

This was the state in which the hospital had been handed over to us. It was a military hospital whose staff had had orders to leave at four o'clock that morning, and they handed the whole hospital with its 270 patients over to us just as it was, and we could do very little towards making it more comfortable for them. The stench of the whole place was horrible, but it was too cold to do more than open the window for a minute or two every now and then. It was no one's fault that things were in such a horrible condition, it was just the force of circumstances and the fortune of war that the place had been taxed far beyond its possible capacities.

All night long the most terribly wounded men were being brought in from the field, some were already dead when they arrived, others had only a few minutes to live; all the rest were very cold and wet and exhausted, and we had nothing to make them comfortable. What a blessing hot-water bottles would have been, but after all there would have been no hot water to fill them with. But the wounded had to be brought in for shelter somewhere, and at least we had a roof over their heads, and hot tea to give them.

At 5 A. M. there came a lull. The tragic procession ceased for a while, and we went to lie down. At seven o'clock we were called again, as another batch of wounded was being brought in.

The shelling had begun again, and was terrific; crash, crash, over our heads the whole time. A clock-tower close to the hospital was demolished and windows broken everywhere. The shells were bursting everywhere in the street, and civilians were being brought in to us severely wounded. A little child was carried in with half its head blown open, and then an old Jewish woman with both legs blown off, and a terrible wound in her chest, who only lived an hour or two. Apparently she suffered no pain, but was most dreadfully agitated, poor old dear, at having lost her wig in the transit. They began bringing in so many that we had to stop civilians being brought in at all, as it was more than we could do to cope with the wounded soldiers who were being brought in all the time.

At midday we went to a hotel for a meal. There was very little food left in Lodz, but they brought what they could. Coming back to the hospital we tried everywhere to get some bread, but there was none to be had anywhere, as all the provision shops were quite empty, and the inhabitants looked miserable and starved, the Jewish population particularly so, though they were probably not among the poorest.

On our way back a shell burst quite close to us in the street, but fortunately no one was injured. These shells make a most horrible screeching scream before bursting, like an animal in pain. Ordinarily I am the most dreadful coward in the world about loud noises. I even hate a thunderstorm , but here somehow the shells were so part of the whole thing that one did not realize that all this was happening to us, one felt rather like a disinterested spectator at a far-off dream. It was probably partly due to want of sleep; one's hands did the work, but one's mind was mercifully numbed, for it was more like hell than anything I can imagine. The never-ending processions of groaning men being brought in on those horrible blood-soaked stretchers, suffering unimagined tortures, the filth, the cold, the stench, the hunger, the vermin, and the squalor of it all, added to one's utter helplessness to do more than very little to relieve their misery, was almost enough to make even Satan weep.

On the third day after our arrival a young Russian doctor and some Russian nurses arrived to relieve us for a few hours, and we most thankfully went to bed. It was not a bed in the ordinary sense, but a wire bedstead that squeaked incessantly at the slightest movement. We were so exhausted that we lay down in all our clothes; but we were very comfortable all the same.

When we woke up we were told that the military authorities had given orders for the patients to be evacuated, and that Red Cross carts were coming all night to take them away to the station, where some ambulance trains awaited them. So we worked hard all night to get the dressings done before the men were sent away, and as we finished each case, he was carried down to the hall to await his turn to go; but it was very difficult as all the time they were bringing in fresh cases just as fast as they were taking the others away, and many had to go off without having had their dressings done at all. The next afternoon we were still taking the wounded in, when we got another order that all the fresh patients were to be evacuated and the hospital closed, as the Russians had decided to retire from Lodz. Again we worked all night, and by ten the next morning we had gotten all the patients away. The stretcher bearers collected all the bedding in the yard to be burnt, the bedsteads were piled high on one another, and we opened all the windows wide to let the clean cold wind blow over everything.

We had all our own dressings and equipment to pack, and were all just about at our last gasp from want of food and sleep, when a very kind Polish lady came and asked us all to sleep at her house. I never looked forward to anything so much in my life as I did to my bed that night. Our hostess simply heaped benefits on us by preparing us each a hot bath in turn. We had not washed or had our clothes off since we came to Lodz, and were covered with vermin which had come to us from the patients. There are three varieties commonly met with: ordinary fleas that no one minds in the least; white insects that are the commonest and live in the folds of one's clothes, whose young are most difficult to find, and who grow middle-aged and very hungry in a single night; and, lastly, the red insects with a good many legs, which are much less numerous but much more ravenous than the other kinds.

After the baths, we sat down to a delicious supper, and were looking forward to a still more delicious night in bed, when a captain arrived and said we must leave at once. We guessed instantly that the Germans must be very near, but that he did not wish us to ask questions, as it seemed very mean to go off ourselves and leave our kind hosts without a word of explanation, though of course we could only obey orders. So we left our unfinished supper and quickly collected our belongings and took them to the hotel where our Red Cross car should have been waiting for us. But the Red Cross authorities had sent off our car with some wounded, which of course was just as it should be, and we were promised another "seechas," which literally translated signifies "immediately," but in Russia means today or tomorrow or not at all.

Nothing can express utter desolation much more nakedly than a Grand Hotel that has been through a week or two's bombardment. Here indeed were the mighty fallen. A large hole was ripped out of the wall of the big restaurant, close to the alcove where the band used to play while the smart people dined. An elaborate wine-list still graced each little table, but coffee made from rye bread crusts mixed with a little chicory was the only drink that a few white-faced waiters who crept about the room like shadows could apologetically offer us. We sat there till nearly 3 A. M., when utterly worn out with physical and mental fatigue, most of us drifted off to sleep where we sat.

In the morning things began to look cheerful. The Germans had still not arrived, our own car turned up, and best of all, we were officially told that every wounded man who was at all transportable had now been successfully removed from Lodz. It was a gigantic task, this evacuation of over 18,000 wounded in four days, and it is incredible that it was done successfully.

It was a most lovely day with a soft blue sky, and all the world bathed in winter sunshine. Shelling had ceased during the night, but began again with terrific force in the morning, and we started off under a perfect hail of shells. There were four German aeroplanes hovering just above us, throwing down bombs at short intervals. The shells aimed at them looked so innocent, like little white puff-balls bursting up in the blue sky. We hoped they would be brought down, but they were too high for that. The bombs were only a little diversion of theirs by the way, as they were really trying to locate the Russian battery, as they were evidently making signals to their own headquarters. Danger always adds a spice to every entertainment, and as the wounded were all out and we had nobody but ourselves to think about, we could enjoy our thrilling departure from Lodz under heavy fire to the uttermost. And I must say I have rarely enjoyed anything more. It was simply glorious spinning along in that car, and we got out safely without anyone being hurt.

We passed through Breeziny, where the tail-end of a battle was going on, and the driver stopped the car for a few minutes so that we could see the men in the trenches. On our way, we passed crowds of terrified refugees hurrying along the road with their few possessions on their backs or in their arms; it reminded me of those sad processions of flying peasants in Belgium, but I think these were mostly much poorer, and had not so much to lose. Just as the sun was setting we stopped and looked back, and the sky was bloody and lurid over the western plain where

CANADIAN ANGELS OF MERCY

Lodz lay. To us it seemed like an ill omen for the unhappy town, but it may be that the Germans took those flaming clouds to mean that even the heavens themselves were illuminated to signal their victory.

Some bread and some pale golden Hungarian Tokay were produced by our host for our refreshment. The latter was delicious, but it must have been much more potent than it looked, for though I only had one small glass of it, I collapsed altogether afterwards, and lay on the floor of the car, and could not move till the lights of Warsaw were in sight. In a few minutes more, we arrived at the Hotel Bristol, and then the Flying Column went to bed at last.[82]

Lodz As It Relates to Canadian Nurses

The Polish front was every bit as brutal as the rest of the western front, and all nurses shared the commonality of facing extremely adverse conditions to which they had to readily adept. The immense dangers were ever present in a war of attrition that measured success by a few metres at a time. The slaughter was incredibly mechanized like no other war, and the medical staff had never encountered such wide-spread carnage, nor been trained in how to handle it.

After the battle, nurse Alice Issacson summed-up the extraordinary implications of this battle and how it would affect the on-going effort in the following diary entry: *Thank God for an imagination, and a quick appreciation! Embellishing the perhaps otherwise commonplace in our daily life with both beauty and pathos! One goes about in the midst of men, intent on daily duties, and yet finding*

---

[82] Retrieved from http://www.gutenberg.org/files/17587/17587-h/pg131

touches of beauty, and sudden expression of the deeper and holier currents in human hearts, that stand out like precious jewels in the somber "sameness" and "commonness" of the day's routine. The war is brutal and unforgiving, but that does not mean we have to lose our humanity in the process.[83]

Over 320,000 men were wounded, captured or killed at Lodz. The nurses there were under some of the heaviest bombardments of the war, and they were commended in a communiqué from a Russian general who summed up their contribution in a telegram sent to the British High Command: *If it were not for the fearless courage of the nurses, many more of our valiant soldiers would have died. They braved great hardships and ceaseless enemy fire to save the lives of countless men. When the roll of honour is called, they should be at the front of the line.*

---

[83] Retrieved from http//www.gutenberg.org/files/17587/17587-h/17587-h.htm

CHAPTER 12
AN ENEMY MORE DEADLY THAN ANY WE SAW
IN THE WAR

Étaples was on the western front and over 100,000 soldiers were being housed in tents and make-shift barracks. Additionally, up to 6500 patients were in the various Étaples hospitals. Within a 20 kilometre area, there were two million soldiers encamped and over six million occupied the trenches along a stretch of land from the English Channel to the Swiss border. The conditions under which all these people lived were an ideal breeding ground for the spread of a respiratory virus.

All these elements were compounded by a complete disregard of proper sanitary procedures by military authorities in charge of the cantonment. Ignoring the admonitions of the medical staff was common place as staff officers were more concerned with combat operations than the safety of the men when it came to sanitary conditions. This led to perilous situations that were created by soldiers who purchased live geese, chickens and ducks. They would slaughter them and leave the carcasses lying all about the camp. This made the entire town a breeding ground for cross species transfer of avian flu.

Within these conditions, the soldiers were timidly anticipatory that the war seemed to be winding down. Yet, many of them would survive battle only to be felled by another war waged against them by a virus. October 1918 would usher in an era that ended man's war against man, but saw the death toll among soldiers rise, not from bombs and bullets, but from a deadly disease that was even greater than the black plague that ravaged Europe in the Middle Ages. Before the disease had run its course, millions of people would die. Twenty out of every 1000 people alive at the time would succumb to the flu. For over four years, healthcare professionals had fought valiantly to keep the broken in mind, body and spirit fit to fight. Now, they would face an enemy greater than any of the armies – an infectious virus.

Most virologists suggest that Étaples was at the very centre of this rapidly mutating virus as early as 1916. Since autopsies were a rarity, it is postulated that many of the soldiers who survived their wounds, but died later in the hospital, may have succumbed as a result of this virus that had led to complications. Once the war ended, these soldiers and medical personnel returned to their home countries, carrying this deadly virus with them.

Although often referred to as the Spanish flu, because the first identifiable case appeared in Spain in early 1918, most scientists categorically ascribe to the theory that it originated Étaples. Nurses in Étaples had been experiencing debilitating fatigue and fevers since March or April of 1916. Many of them were sent back to England for rest and recuperation, as it was erroneously assumed they were just suffering from extreme exhaustion as a result of overwork. However, they may have had an early form of the flu which would eventually mutate into a much more deadly virus.

In Canada, over 60,000 people died from this virulent strain of influenza. In some Quebec and Labrador remote villages, the entire population was wiped out. Nurses, who had returned home hoping for some rest from the rigors of war, were once again faced with overwhelming dependence on their courage and devotion to serve those who needed them.

It is assumed the first flu case in Canada was on 9 September 1918, when nine American soldiers who had been ill died in Quebec City. Within days, it had spread to Ontario and then to the prairies as troop trains carrying returning soldiers headed west. Some towns even refused to allow train passengers to disembark. By 9 October, 2500 cases had been reported in Brantford, Ontario. Before long, public meetings were banned. Schools, universities and public facilities closed, and people who had to go out, did so with great trepidation and most wore masks.

Again, the vanguard for those who fell ill were the tireless nurses who refused to give into despair and could be found ministering aid day and night in hospitals, homes and make-shift facilities set-up to care for the afflicted. They did all this with total disregard for their own safety and welfare.

Aboriginal communities, especially in the north, were particularly hard hit. On the Peace River Reserve, where the majority of residents lived in log cabins or tepees, 85% of the residents died. An Ontario nurse paddled down the Kapuskasing River to take the only two Aboriginal children who survived a flu outbreak in a small village to a district aid station.

Many communities ran out of coffins, and in some rural snow-bound areas, there was no time, and in some cases, no able-bodied men to bury the dead, so the corpses were placed on the roofs of cabins to keep them from being eaten by wild animals. In these far-flung communities, nurses were often the only medical help available.

Today, it is difficult for Canadians with the finest healthcare system in the world to imagine, at this time in

Canada there was no guaranteed free medical care for all Canadians; consequently, most people simply could not afford the care they needed. For that reason, the majority of people were nursed at home. Unselfishly, nurses all over Canada volunteered to work extra hours outside hospitals free-of-charge. When their hospital duties were over, you could find them going from home-to-home caring for the afflicted.

Like so much of the world today, there were those in 1918 whose greed took precedence over compassion, as the profit motive, as it often does, reared its ugly, sinister head even in Canada. Some women began to pose as nurses and were charging as much as $25 a day to tend to the sick in their homes, while the real nurses were working for $2 a day. Disinfectants suddenly escalated in price at many stores from 50 cents a pound to as much as $10 a pound. Mask prices shot up from 5 cents to over $1. Because people feared the use of tin cups for drinking, paper cup manufacturers and retailers jacked-up the prices over 1000%. Other entrepreneurs hawked cinnamon, alcohol, tobacco and turpentine as cures. Meanwhile, as the hucksters lined their pockets with ill-gotten gain, the nurses methodically went about their duties dispensing care and compassion.

As the soldiers returned home from the horrors of war, they were now faced with an equally virulent killer every bit as deadly as an enemy gun, bayonet or bomb. When they would get off a troop train, they often found their mothers, fathers, wives and children unable to touch them for fear of contracting the deadly virus. The irony of the situation can be illustrated with the case of Canada's youngest recipient of the Victoria Cross, 18 year old Airman Alan McLeod of Manitoba, who survived many air battles, including one with the red baron, only to be fatally struck down by the flu upon his return home.

One nurse, Annie Sheldon, who worked at the North Battleford, Saskatchewan Hospital was noted for her intense commitment to her patients and refusal to leave the hospital and go home to her husband and children. Ultimately, every nurse became infected and only one doctor and Sheldon were left to care for hundreds of patients. Using disinfectant on themselves every few hours and never going without a mask, the two of them managed to avoid contracting the flu.

While the larger cities were better equipped to handle the vast number of cases, the rural areas were ill-prepared and lacked the antibiotics needed tocombat the disease. Nurses who had served so valiantly in the war were the heart and soul of the battle against this raging epidemic. Leaving one war behind, they had come home to fight another war. It is estimated that 50,000,000 to 100,000,000[84] people died worldwide, and many doctors and nurses succumbed as a result of their devotion to serving those in peril. One nurse in Nova Scotia said, "we left many horrors behind in the bombed out cities and fields of Flanders, only to come home and find an enemy more deadly than any we saw in the war."

---

[84] Retrieved from http://www.oddee.com/item_90608.aspx

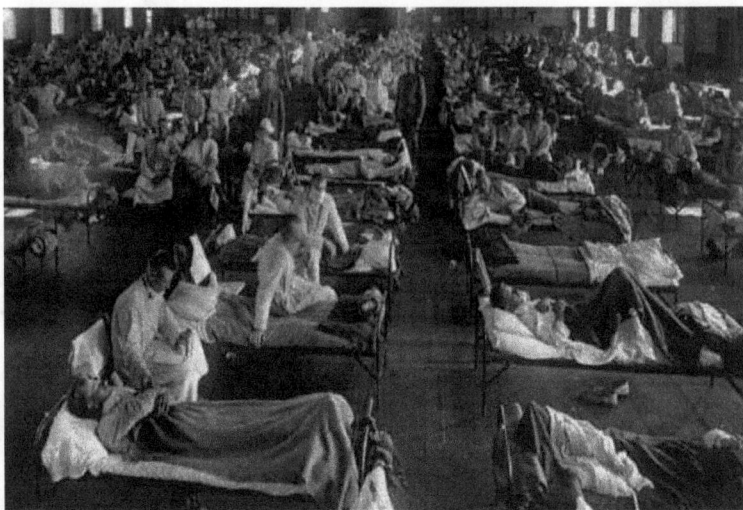

Canadian Hospitals Were so Overwhelmed That They Had
to Set-up Special Quarters in Warehouses, Gyms and
Vacant Buildings (Above Photo Taken in 1918)[85]

---

[85] Retrieved from http://www.ca?CTVNews/20110919/spanish-flu-out
break-study-110919/

EPILOGUE

Facts on Canada's Nursing Sisters[86]

- Canada's Nursing Sisters have a proud legacy of military service that dates back as far as 1885, when for the first time, Canadian nurses were part of the medical and surgical team deployed to care for soldiers wounded during the North-West Rebellion.
- The first nurses to serve in war were women who belonged to religious orders – hence, the designation of "Nursing Sister" and the traditional white veil.
- Nursing Sisters also provided medical service as part of the Royal Canadian Dragoons contingent that was sent, in 1898, to the Klondike to assist the Northwest Mounted Police during the gold rush.
- Prince Edward Island's Georgina Fane Pope, one of Canada's pioneer Nursing Sisters, who served in the South African war, trained in New York City at Bellevue Hospital's Nightingale School. The school was named for the world's most well-known nurse, Florence Nightingale, of Great Britain.
- A total of 3,141 Canadian nurses volunteered their services during the Great War of 1914-1918. At first, the army medical units were set up in hospitals away from the action. Eventually, however, Casualty Clearing Stations were set up, close to the front lines. It was at these stations that the ambulances would deliver the injured who

---

[86] Information compiled from Canadian Department of Veterans Affairs

received early stage assessment and, as a result, obtained quicker and more effective treatment.

- During the First World War, 47 to 53 Nursing Sisters gave their lives: Thought not complete, the death list included six killed or mortally wounded (of which three died in the deliberate bombing of the military hospital in Étaples, France); 15 died at sea, with the sinking of the hospital ship, *Llandovery Castle*; 15 died of disease; and seven died from wounds or illness back home, in Canada.
- During the Second World War, Canada's nursing service was expanded to all three branches of the military – the Navy, the Army and the Air Force – with each branch having its own distinctive uniform and working dress, while all wore the white veil.
- A total of 4,473 Nursing Sisters served during the Second World War, many of whom found themselves within range of enemy guns. At first, almost all field hospital units were set up under canvas tents, many of which later would move to bombed-out or abandoned buildings.
- During the Battle of the Atlantic, Canada had two navy hospital ships, the *Letitia* and the *Lady Nelson*, both of which were staffed by army Sisters. The navy Sisters served on naval bases on both coasts of Canada.
- The nursing service of the Royal Canadian Air Force was not established until November of 1940. With more than 100 station hospitals having been constructed, the demand for additional Nursing Sisters increased. Some were trained in air evacuation, 12 served in Newfoundland flying air-sea rescue missions, and 66 went overseas.
- During the Second World War, the nursing service also included four special branches:

The Physiotherapists, Occupational Therapists, Dieticians and Home Sisters. In addition, there were Sisters who served on the hospital trains that returned the wounded to destinations across Canada.

- During United Nations operations in Korea, in the 1950s, Nursing Sisters served in both Korea and Japan. Others flew air evacuation with casualties back to Canada. Another specialty, which 5 RCAF Nursing Sisters joined, was the Para-Rescue Service. When the cease-fire came into effect, the Sisters tended to the newly released prisoners of war, helping them to regain their health.
- In more recent times, Nursing Officers (as they are now called) have served in the Gulf War, and in peace-keeping missions in Bosnia-Herzegovina, Rwanda and Somalia.

A Final Word

World War I and the flu epidemic were defining forces in the development of nursing as a respected and revered profession. No longer were nurses looked upon with disdain and disrespect. The public and other medical professionals began to realize the vital role nurses play in patient care. The great confluence of events between 1885 and 1918 solidified the sisterhood of those called to this exalted profession. Today's nurses can look to these women as role models who paved the way for this noble endeavour.

Canadian soldiers returning from the war played a significant role in the new-found respect for nurses by the public, as their stories of the heroic and compassionate care they received from "their angels of mercy" were a frequent topic of discussion throughout Canada. Not only were the soldiers who served praised and venerated by the public, but so were the nurses.

Nurses contributions to the war effort set a precedence for women and their role in society, from which they refused to regress. They may have made up only a small portion of those who served, but their impact reached far beyond their numbers. It was the success of nurses in World War I that made women in Canada begin to realize that they no longer had to submit to a subservient role. Though the struggle would be long and arduous, women had found a determination they never had before, and it was the nurses who helped solidify this determination that would lead to a more equalitarian society. For that, we must be eternally grateful to the Canadian angels of mercy who served in times of peril.

The End

NON-FOOTNOTED BOOK AND JOURNAL REFERENCES

Abel-Smith B. (1960). A History of the Nursing Profession. London, UK: Heineman Publishing.

Andrews, M.E., Stewart, N.J., Pitblado, J.R., Morgan, D.G., D'Arcy, C., & Forbes, D. (2005). Registered Nurses Working Alone in Rural and Remote Canada. *Canadian Journal of Nursing Research*, 37:1, pp.14-33.

Baker, M. (1983). The Development of the Office of a Permanent Medical Health Officer for St. John's Newfoundland, 1826 – 1905. *HSTC Bulletin*, 7:2, pp. 98-105.

Baly, M. (1986). Florence Nightingale and the Nursing Legacy. London, UK: Croom-Helm Publishing.

Boyer, Y. (2003). The International Right to Health for Indigenous Peoples in Canada. *National Aboriginal Health Organization & The Native Law Centre*, Ottawa/Saskatchewan.

Canadian Institute for Health Information (CIHI). (2002). Supply and Distribution of Registered Nurses in Canada, 2000. Ottawa, Ontario.

Clint, M. (1934). Our Bit: Memories of War Service by a Canadian Nursing Sister. Montreal: Quebec. Barwick Publishing.

Davis A. (2005). An Open Letter to the International Community Asking What Are We Going to do About It?

International Council of Nurses. Retrieved from www.icn.ch/INR/comment-inr_466.pdf.

Directorate of History. Department of National Defence. Subject Files – Statistics, Ottawa.

Gibbon, J.& Mathewson, M. (1947). Three Centuries of Canadian Nursing. Toronto, Ontario: The McMillan Company.

Hogan W. (1986). Pathways of Mercy in Newfoundland, 1924-1984. St. Johns, Newfoundland: Harry Cuff Publishing.

MacPherson, K. (1982). Nurses and Nursing in Early Twentieth Century- Halifax. MA Thesis, Dalhousie University.

McPherson, K. (1996). Bedside Manners: The Transformation of Canadian Nursing, 1900-1990. Toronto, Ontario: Oxford University Press.

Mary Southcott File (1980). *Botanique du Canada Bulletin.* 13:2, pp.17-32.

Nevit, J. (1978). White Caps and Black Hands in Newfoundland to 1934. St. John's, Newfoundland: Jesperson Press.

Nicholson, G. (1975). Canada's Nursing Sisters. Toronto, Ontario: Samuels.

Probationer's Register (1909). *The Nursing Mirror.* 9 October 1909, p.22.

Reverby, S. (1982). The Nursing Disorder: A Critical History of Hospital Nursing Relationship. Ph. Dissertation, Boston University.

Royal Commission Testimony of Mary Southcott and Bertha Forsey (1915). Annual Reports of the General Hospital.

Schnarch, B. (2004). Ownership, Control, Access and Possession (OCAP) on Self Determination Applied to Research: A Critical Analysis of Contemporary First Nations Research and Some Options for First Nations Communities in Canada. *NAHO Journal of Aboriginal Health,* 1:1.

Some Pertinent Questions. *The Canadian.* 1943:39, pp. 269-27.

Ustun, B. & Jakob, R. (2005). Re-Defining Health. Retrieved from http://www.who.int.bulletin-board/83/ustin

Wesley-Esquimaux C. & Smolewski, M. (2004). Historic Trauma and Aboriginal Healing. Retrieved from www.ahf.english/historic_trauma.pdf

Wilton, G. (1918). Our Time In Hell. Kent, UK. Kent Press.

Wilson-Simmie, K. (1981). Lights Out: A Canadian Nursing Sister's Tale. Belleville, Ontario: Mika Publishing.

World Health Organization, (1999). The World Health Organization: Making a Difference. Retrieved from http://www.whr/1999/en/whr99_99.

NON-FOOTNOTED WEB SITES

Aboriginal Health Nursing

http://www.indarticles.com/p/articles/mi_qa3911/is_19991
2/ai_n8870761/

Encyclopedia

http://www.nationsencyclopedia.com/economies/Americas/
Canada.html

General Nursing

http://www.contemporarynurse.com/archives/vol/22/issue/2
/article/749/nursing-indigenous-peoples-and-cultural-
safety
http://ruralnursing.unbc.ca/reports/study/Aboriginal_Report
_FINAL.pdf (Nursing in Remote and Rural Canada)
*International Council of Nurses: Nursing and Development
Policy Background Paper*, (2000). International Council of
Nurses. Retrieved from http://www.icn.ch/policy_paper1

Nursing – World War I Specific

http://pw20c.mcmaster.ca/case-study/angels-mercy-canada-
s-nursing-sisters-world-war-i-and-ii
www.navalandmilitarymuseum.org/resource_pages/unsung
_women/rcn_first_women
http://www.trentu.ca/admin/library/archives/fnursesandww
1.htm
http://www.collectionscanada.gc.ca/military/025002-6070-
e.html
http://www.maureenduffus.com/battlefront-nurses.html

http://www.en.wikipedia.org/wiki/Military_history_of_Can ada_during_World_War_I
http://archives.queensu.ca/Exhibits/archres/wwi-intro/women.html
http://www.veterans.gc.ca/eng/feature/hongkong/hkbios/nu rsingsis
http://www.collectionscanada.gc.ca/nursing-sisters/index-e.html
http://4yearsofww1.info/
http://ufcw141nurses.org/nurse_history.htm
http://www.cahn-achn.ca/pdf/Archival%20Resource%20Guide.pdf
http://nlc-bnc.ca/firstworldwar/025005-2500-e.html
http://www.lac-bac.gc.ca/nursing-sisters/025013-1000-e.html
http://www.health.uottawa.ca/nursinghistory/nhru_staff_ct. htm
http://www.spartacus.schoolnet.co.uk/REVhistoryFWW3.h tm
http://www.trentu.ca/admin/library/archives/fnursesand1.ht m

Statistics Canada

http://www12.statcan.ca

9 780987 972804